Gymnastics Journal
& Meet Survival Guide

RIK FEENEY

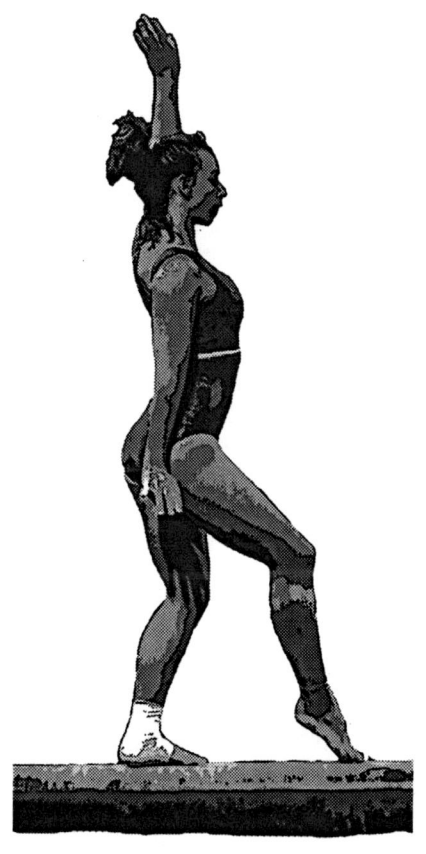

Richardson Publishing
Altamonte Springs, Florida

Gymnastics Journal & Meet Survival Guide
Rik Feeney

Richardson Publishing
PO Box 162115
Altamonte Springs, FL 32716

© 2007 by Richardson Publishing
All Rights Reserved.
Printed in the USA.

info@gymnasticstrainingtips.com
www.gymnasticstrainingtips.com

ISBN: 978-0-9637991-7-3
LCCN: 2007925121

No part of this publication may be reproduced, stored in a retrieval system, or transmitted, in any form or by any means, electronic, mechanical, photocopying, recording, or otherwise, without the prior permission of Richardson Publishing.

DISCLAIMER

This book is written and intended to be used as a guide only. The publisher and author are not engaged in the profession of rendering any form of legal, technical, or medical advice. If for any reason legal, technical or medical advice is necessary, you should seek out qualified professionals.

The purpose of this book is to provide a recorded history of each athlete's competitive experience for future review and reminiscence. Any material supplied to educate the athlete about the competitive experience should be viewed as "suggestions" only with the athlete's personal coach providing the specific guidelines for any and all competitions.

Every effort has been made to provide complete and accurate information on this subject. Readers of this book are strongly advised to obtain guidance and instruction from USAG Safety Certified Coaches.

Any activity, especially one with a high degree of motion, rotation, and height, many times in an inverted (upside-down) position, carries with it a greater potential for injury than normal daily activity. Landing on the head or neck could cause serious and irreparable harm with the potential for fatal consequences to the individual. For this reason, it is advised / demanded that you seek initial training from a Safety Certified gymnastics or cheer coach before using this material for any other purpose than a diary or journal.

The author and Richardson Publishing shall have neither liability nor responsibility to any person or entity with respect to any injury, loss, or damage caused or alleged to be caused directly or indirectly by the information contained in this book.

Illustrations created by: Rik Feeney

This journal belongs to:

Name: _____

USAG #: _____

Team: _____

Parent's
E-mail: _____

Lost Notice

If this book is found wandering by itself, lost at a gym meet, dropped in an airport, or in anyway separated from its owner, please send a note to the email address listed above. At the very least, your reward will be my undying thanks!

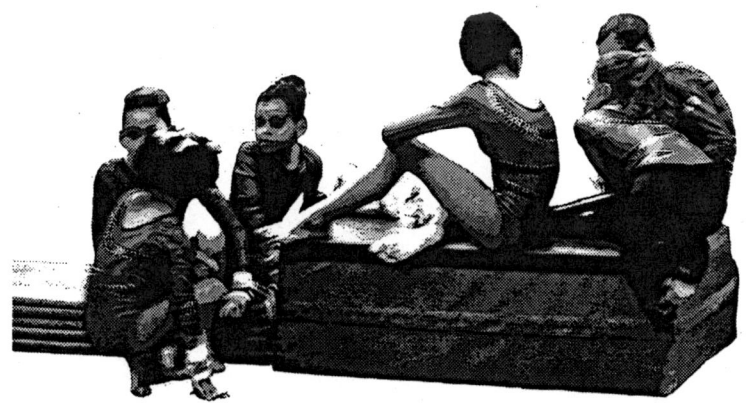

"It's not enough to be good, if you have the ability to be better.

It is not enough to be very good if you have the ability to be great." [1]

- Alberta Lee Cox, grade 8

---

[1] Warner, Carolyn. Treasury of Women's Quotations. Englewood Cliffs, NJ: Prentice Hall, 1992.

Introduction

Pictures and videos are great but not nearly as accessible and personal as a journal written and created by you. This is your journal, a personal record of your experiences as a competitive gymnast.

You are the author of this book, so there is no right or wrong way to develop the material. Several writing prompts are suggested[2], which you are free to use or cross out and use the page for an entirely different reason. It's your book!

The general idea is to record your experience as a competitor from novice to advanced, from a compulsory to optional level gymnast. A new world of experience awaits you at each level. Use this journal to record every thrilling moment!

Answer the questions / prompts with as much or as little detail as you choose. Also included are several special activity pages with lots of fun things to do to and from competitions.

You can personalize this book to make it reflect your tastes, quirks, and personality – or not, the choice is yours. This is your private journal and meet survival guide – for your eyes only, or anyone you specifically give permission.

Someday, maybe that day is today, you can look back and see the person you were as you began your career as a competitive gymnast. You can reminisce alone, share it with friends, or inspire your own children to reach for their goals and learn from your experience.

Good luck. Have a great competitive gymnastics season!

---

[2] Additional notes and ideas for this journal are available online at www.GymnasticsTrainingTips.com.

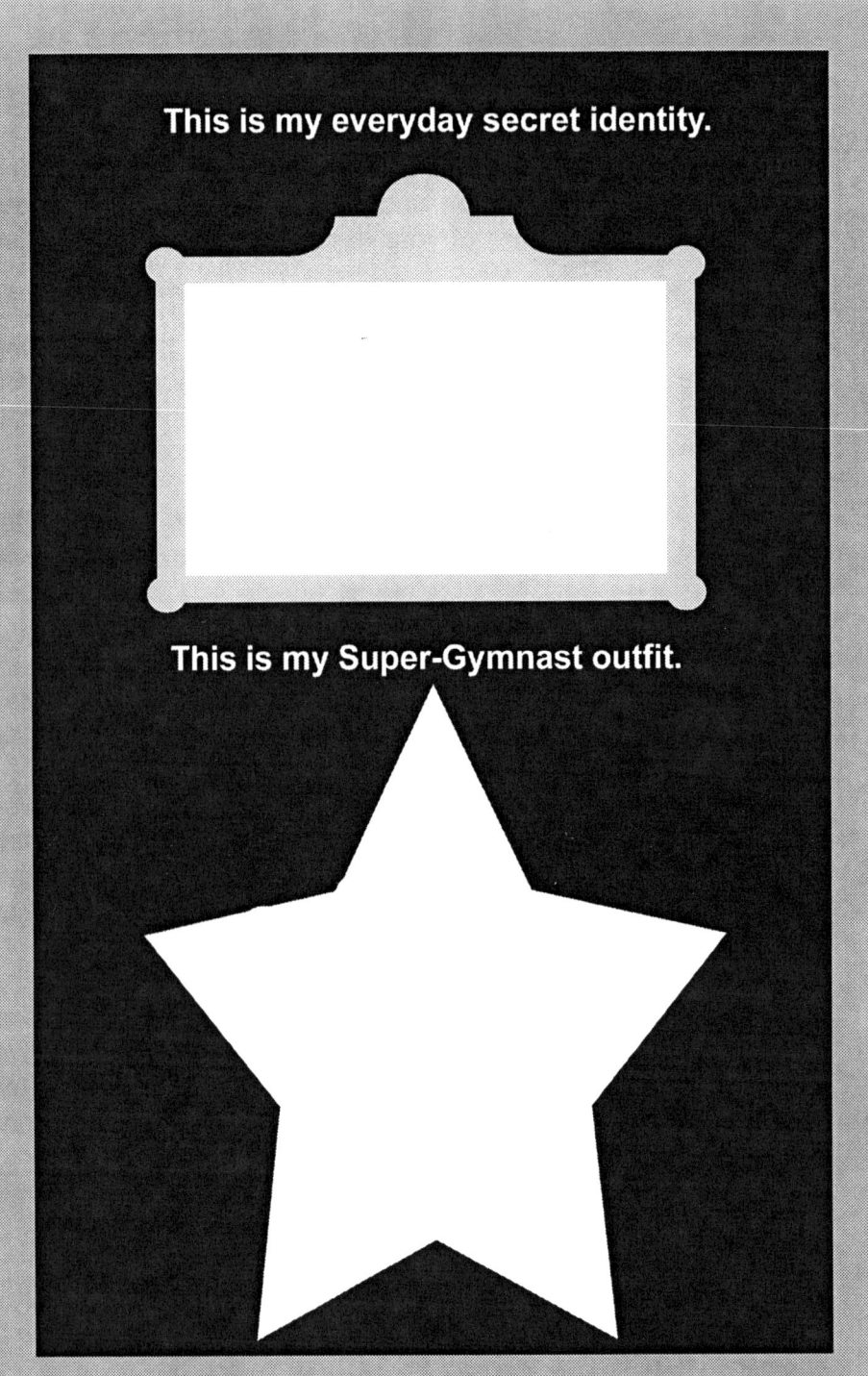

MY FAVORITES PAGE

(My favorite)

Song: _____

Band: _____

TV Show: _____

Movie: _____

Book: _____

Actor: _____

Actress: _____

Gymnastics Event: _____

Hobby: _____

Subject in School: _____

Teacher: _____

Color: _____

Clothes: _____

Snack: _____

Fun Photos

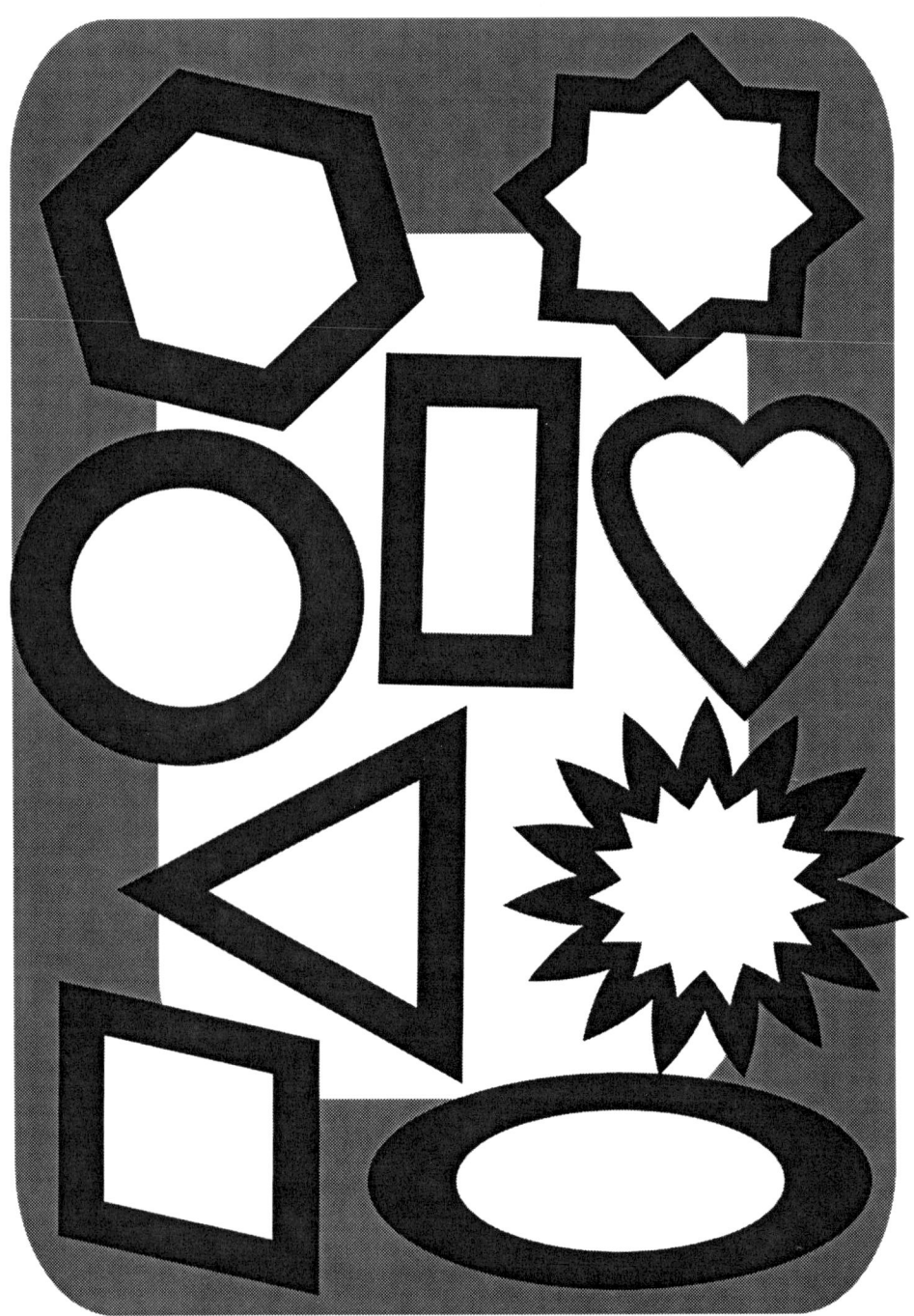

Fun photos

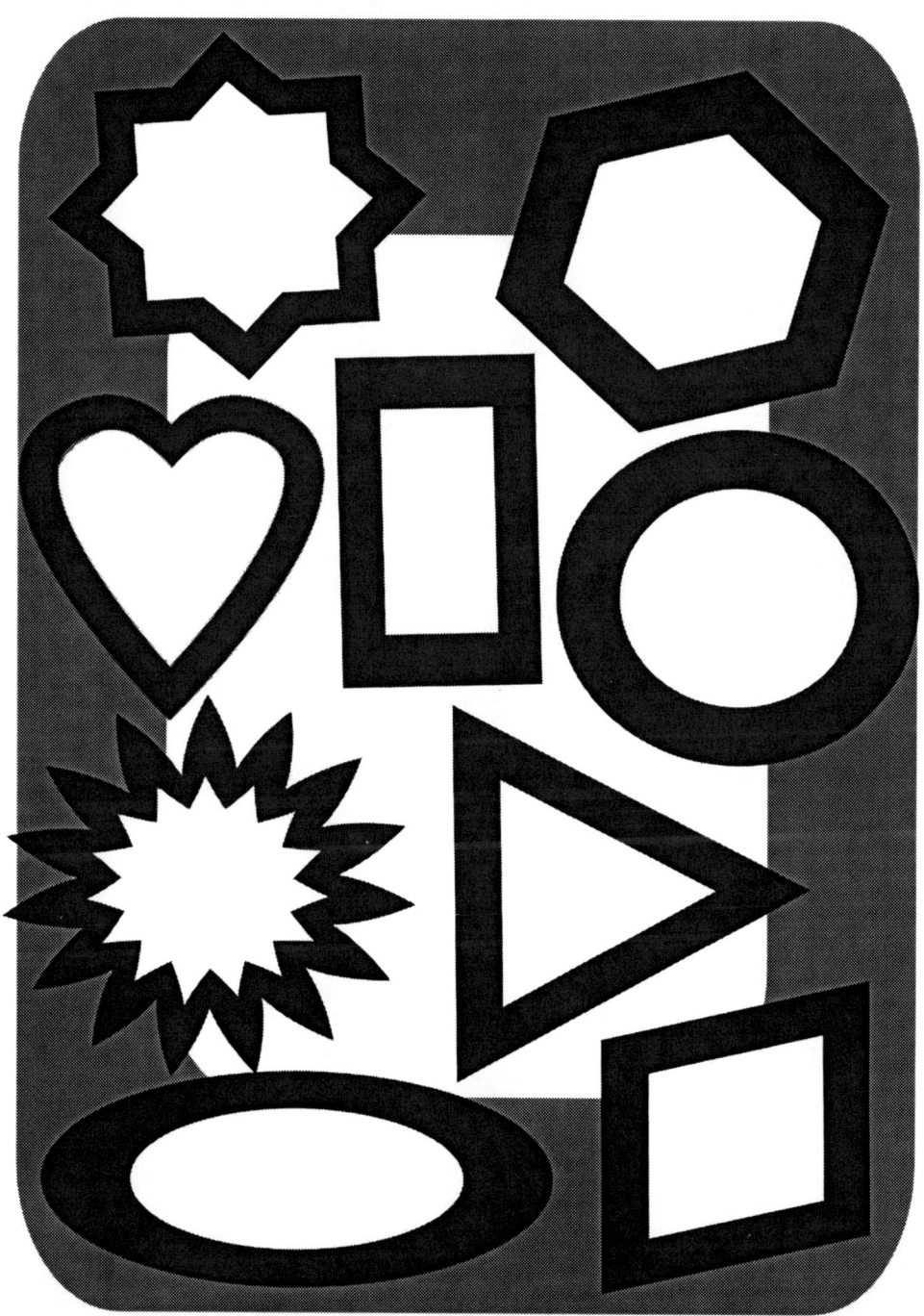

Gymnastics Journal & Meet Survival Guide

Month: **Year:**

Monday	Tuesday	Wednesday	Thursday	Friday	Saturday	Sunday

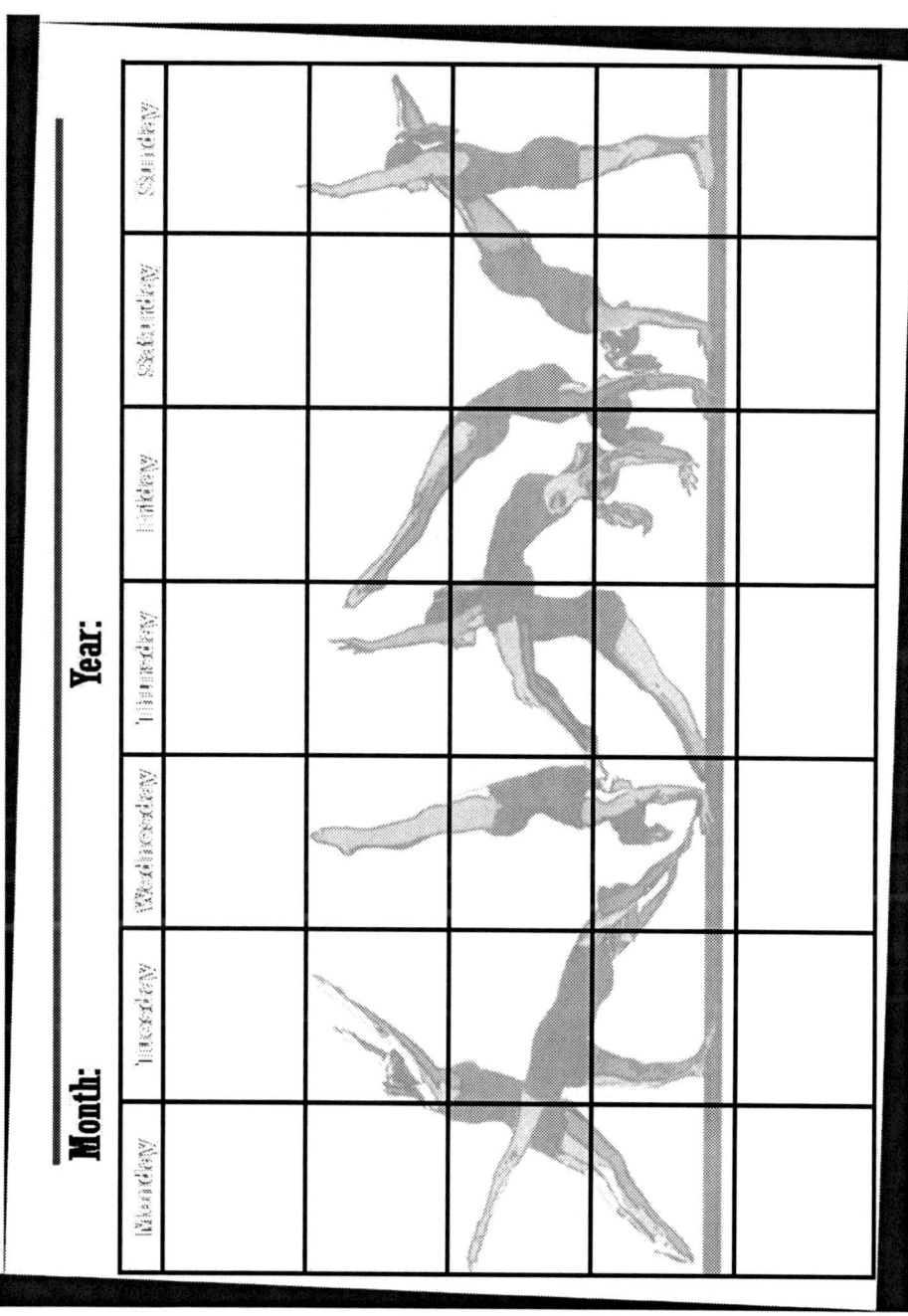

Gymnastics Journal & Meet Survival Guide

Month: _____ **Year:** _____

Monday	Tuesday	Wednesday	Thursday	Friday	Saturday	Sunday

Month: _____ Year: _____

Monday	Tuesday	Wednesday	Thursday	Friday	Saturday	Sunday

Month: _____ Year: _____

Monday	Tuesday	Wednesday	Thursday	Friday	Saturday	Sunday

Month: _____ **Year:** _____

Monday	Tuesday	Wednesday	Thursday	Friday	Saturday	Sunday

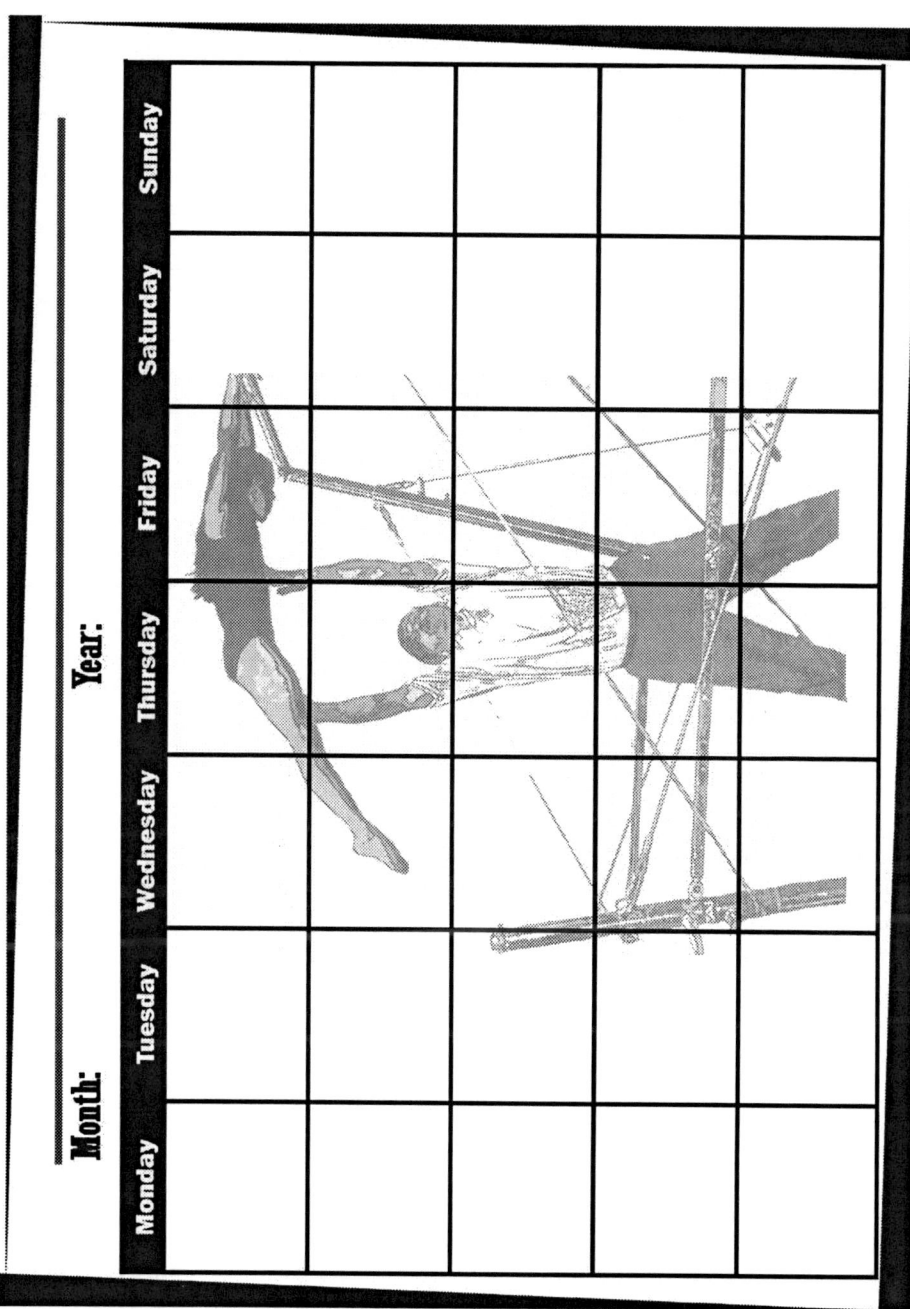

Gymnastics Journal & Meet Survival Guide

Month: _____ **Year:** _____

Monday	Tuesday	Wednesday	Thursday	Friday	Saturday	Sunday

Gymnastics Journal & Meet Survival Guide

Month: _____ **Year:** _____

Monday	Tuesday	Wednesday	Thursday	Friday	Saturday	Sunday

Gymnastics Journal & Meet Survival Guide

Month:			Year:			
Monday	Tuesday	Wednesday	Thursday	Friday	Saturday	Sunday

Month: **Year:**

Monday	Tuesday	Wednesday	Thursday	Friday	Saturday	Sunday

Gymnastics Journal & Meet Survival Guide

Month: _____ **Year:** _____

Monday	Tuesday	Wednesday	Thursday	Friday	Saturday	Sunday

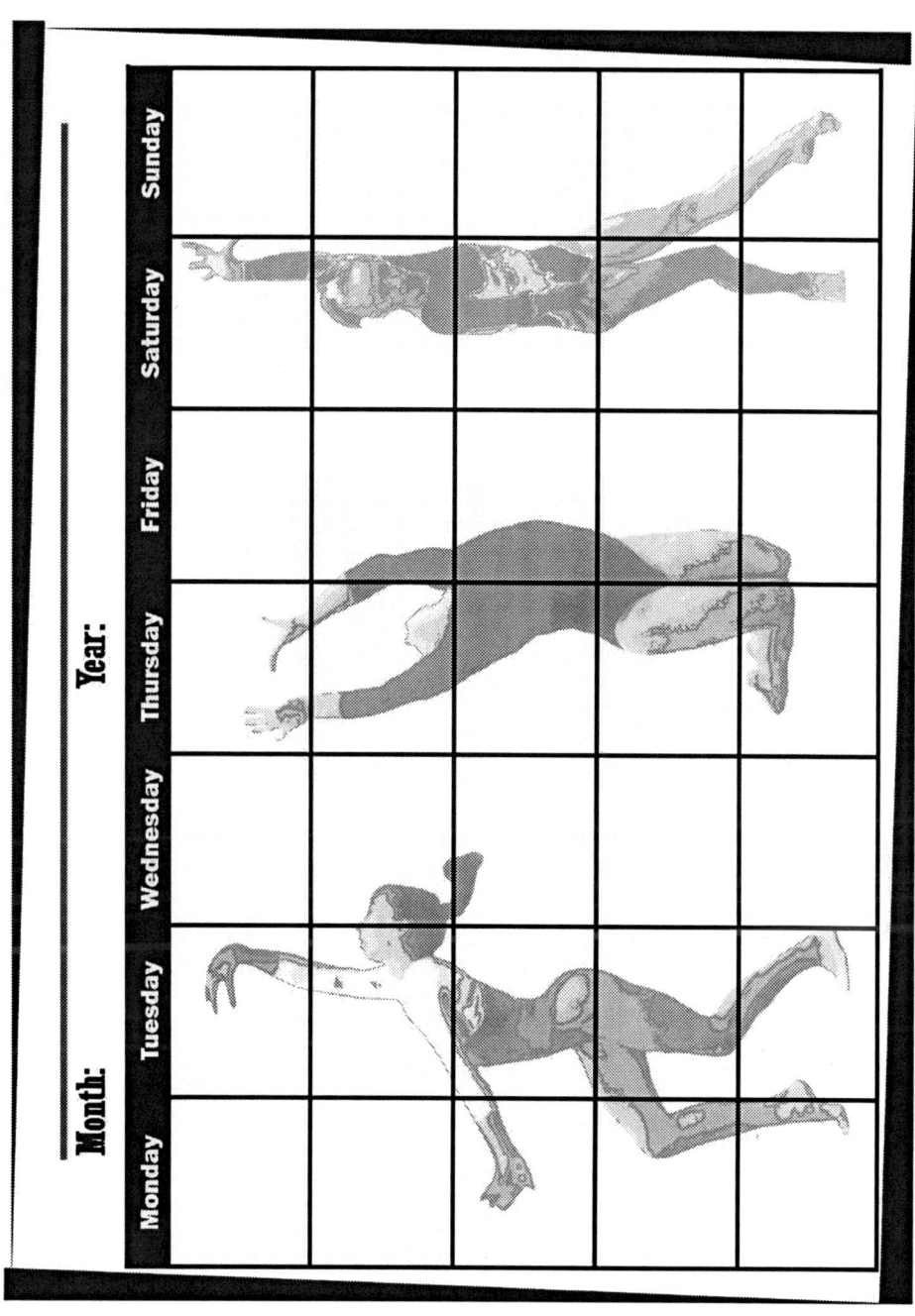

My world

(Make a collage that includes pictures, drawings, funny sayings, stickers – anything that represents your world right now.)

Journal Prompts

Following are questions you can use (or not) to start journal entries (on the blank pages provided directly after these prompts).

- ☐ I started gymnastics because…

- ☐ I wanted to be on the team and compete because…

- ☐ This is what my coach looks like:

- ☐ My coach's favorite sayings are…

- ☐ My best friends on the team this year are…

- ☐ The night before a meet I am …

- ☐ The thing I like most about competition is…

- ☐ The thing I would most like to change about competition is…

- ☐ My favorite event is _____ and the reason why is…

- ☐ The event I need to improve most is _____ and the reason why is…

- ☐ I am really good at…

- ☐ The best thing in my goody bag this season was…

- ☐ Just before competing for the very first time I felt like…

- ☐ The thing I remember most about this season is…

- ☐ When my friends at school ask about gymnastics, I tell them…

- ☐ My favorite thing to eat before a meet is…
- ☐ My least favorite event is the…
- ☐ My current goal in gymnastics is to…
- ☐ The most important thing I learned from my coach is…
- ☐ The most important thing I would tell a new gymnast is…
- ☐ My top ten most favorite things about gymnastics are…
- ☐ My favorite thing to do after a meet is…
- ☐ Use 10 or more single word adjectives to describe yourself as a competitive gymnast.
- ☐ List your positive traits (behaviors, qualities, characteristics) as a competitive gymnast.
- ☐ Make a list of things you would like to improve about yourself as a gymnast.
- ☐ Describe the perfect gymnastics meet.
- ☐ Who is the first person you want to call and tell all about the meet when it is over?
- ☐ What do you say to yourself after a particularly good meet?
- ☐ What do you say to yourself after a particularly bad meet? *(Can you improve your self-talk so everything you say internally helps you grow and get better?)*

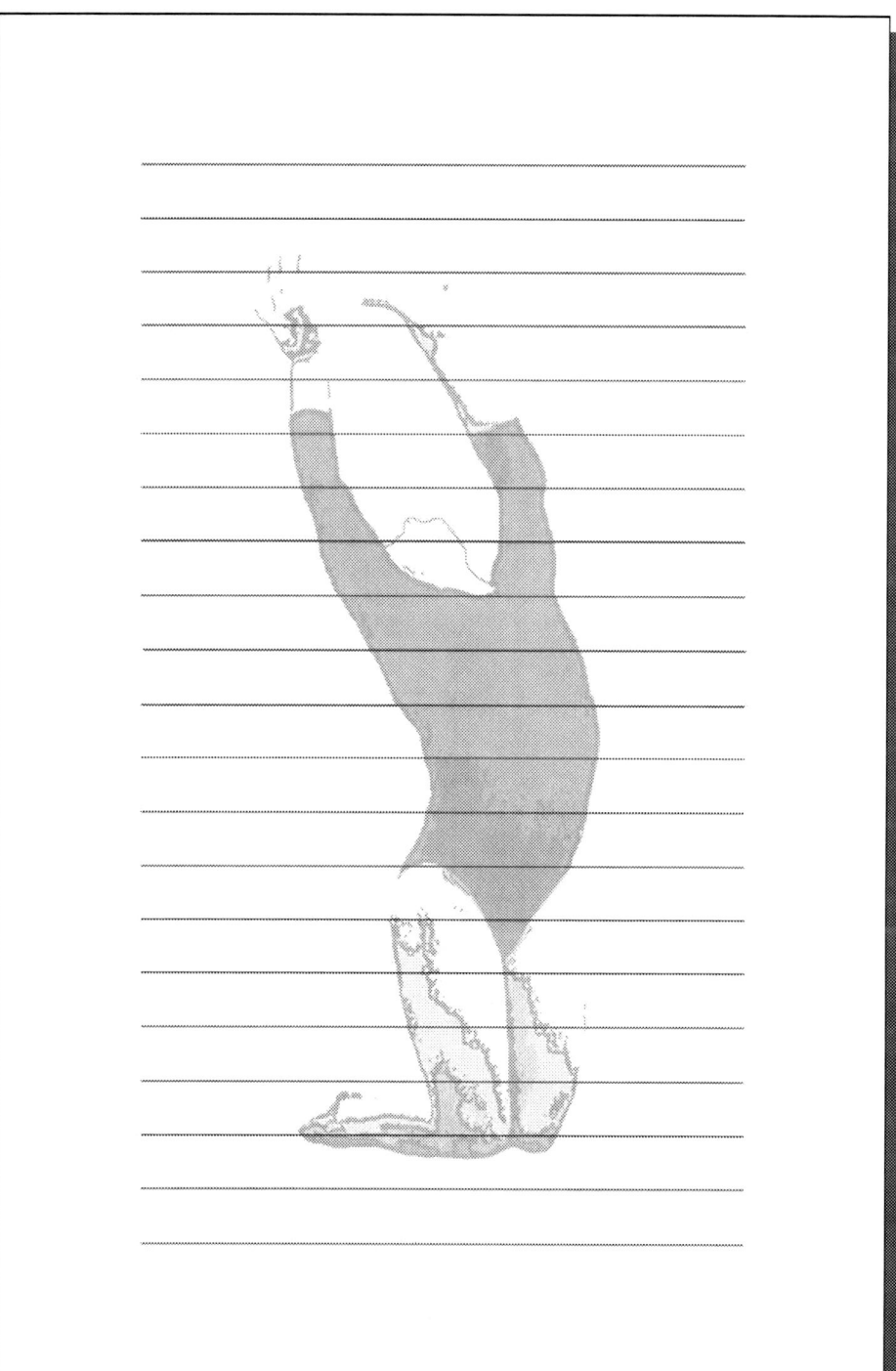

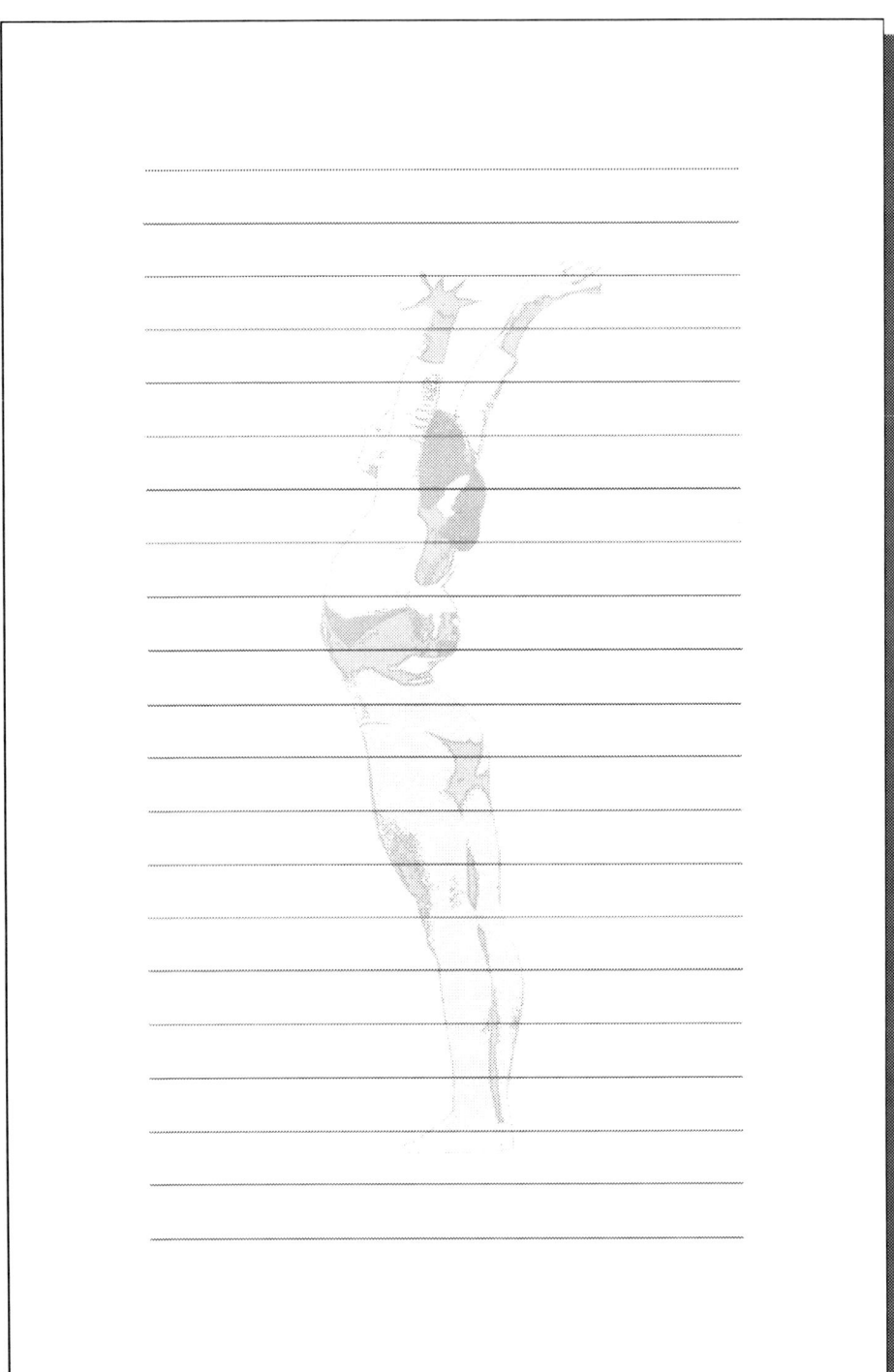

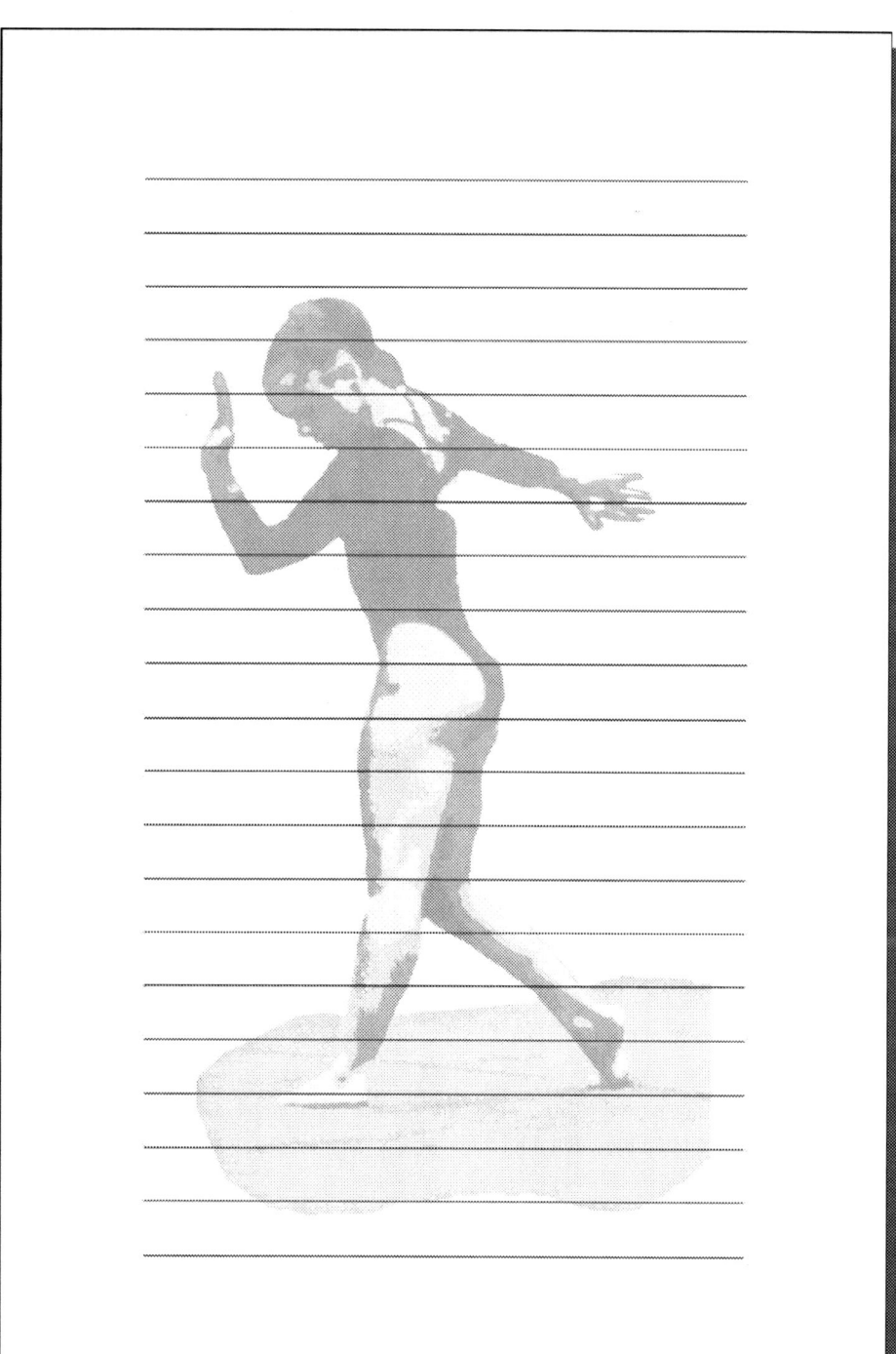

Gymnastics Journal & Meet Survival Guide

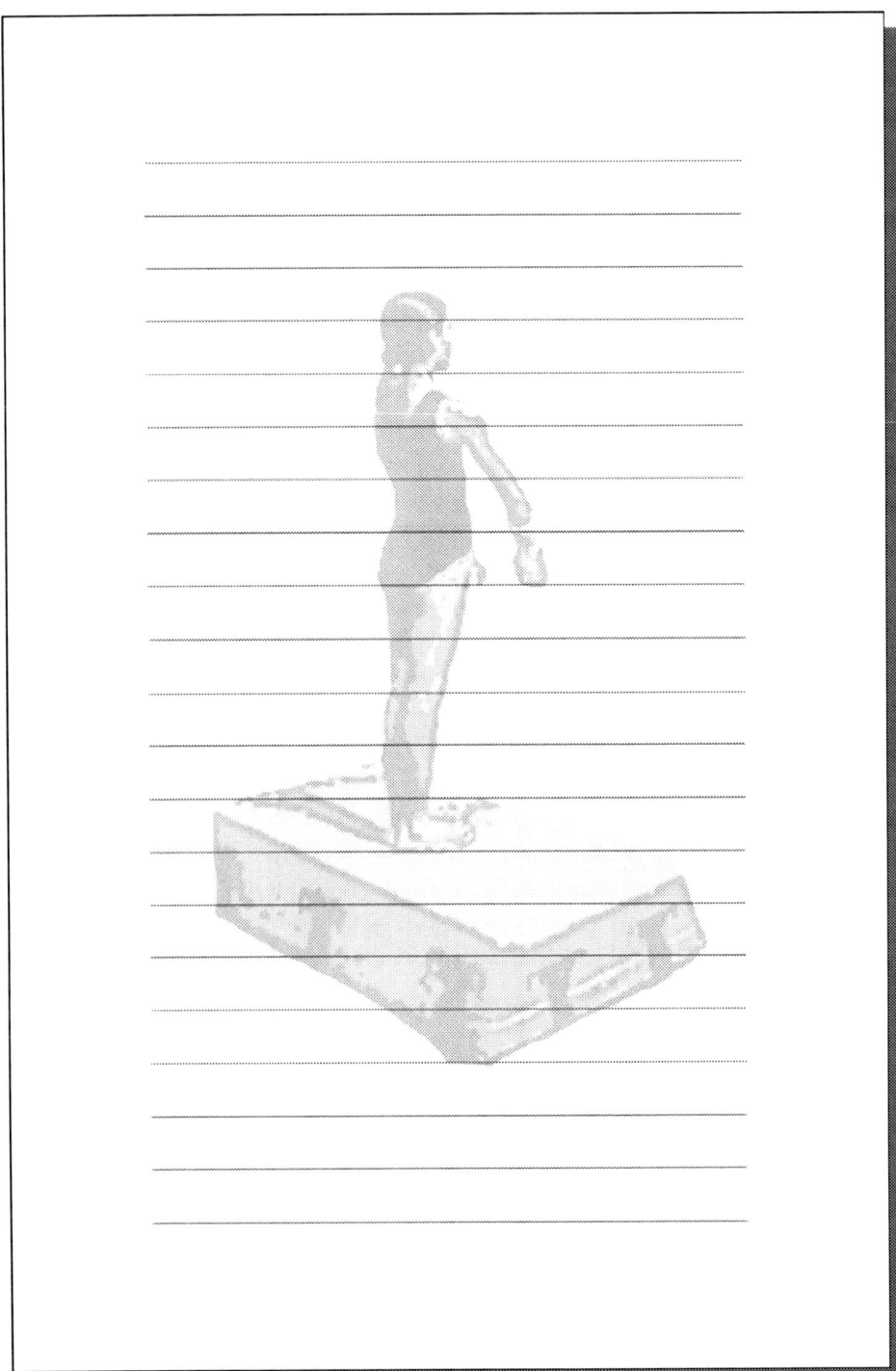

Gymnastics Journal & Meet Survival Guide

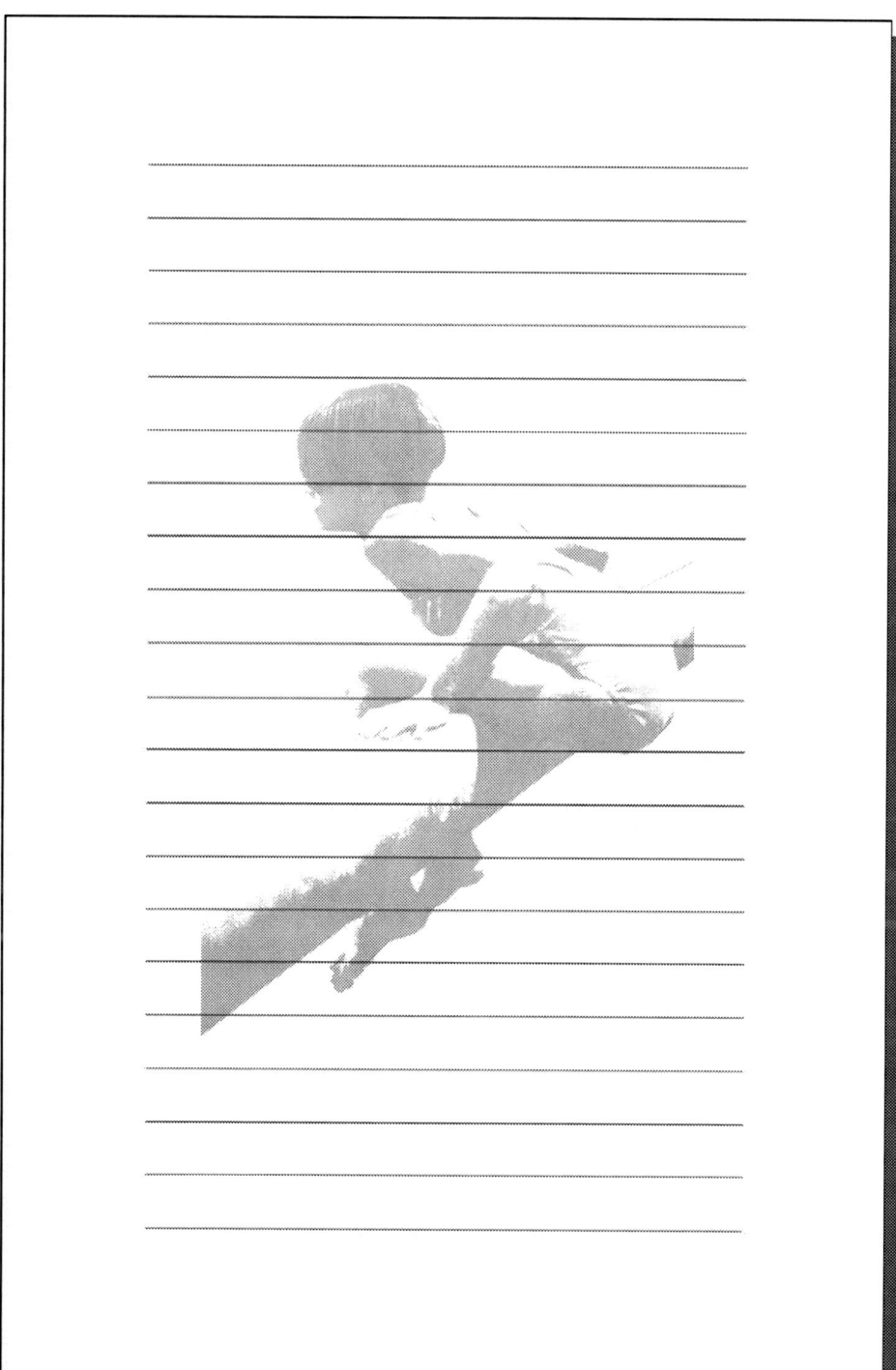

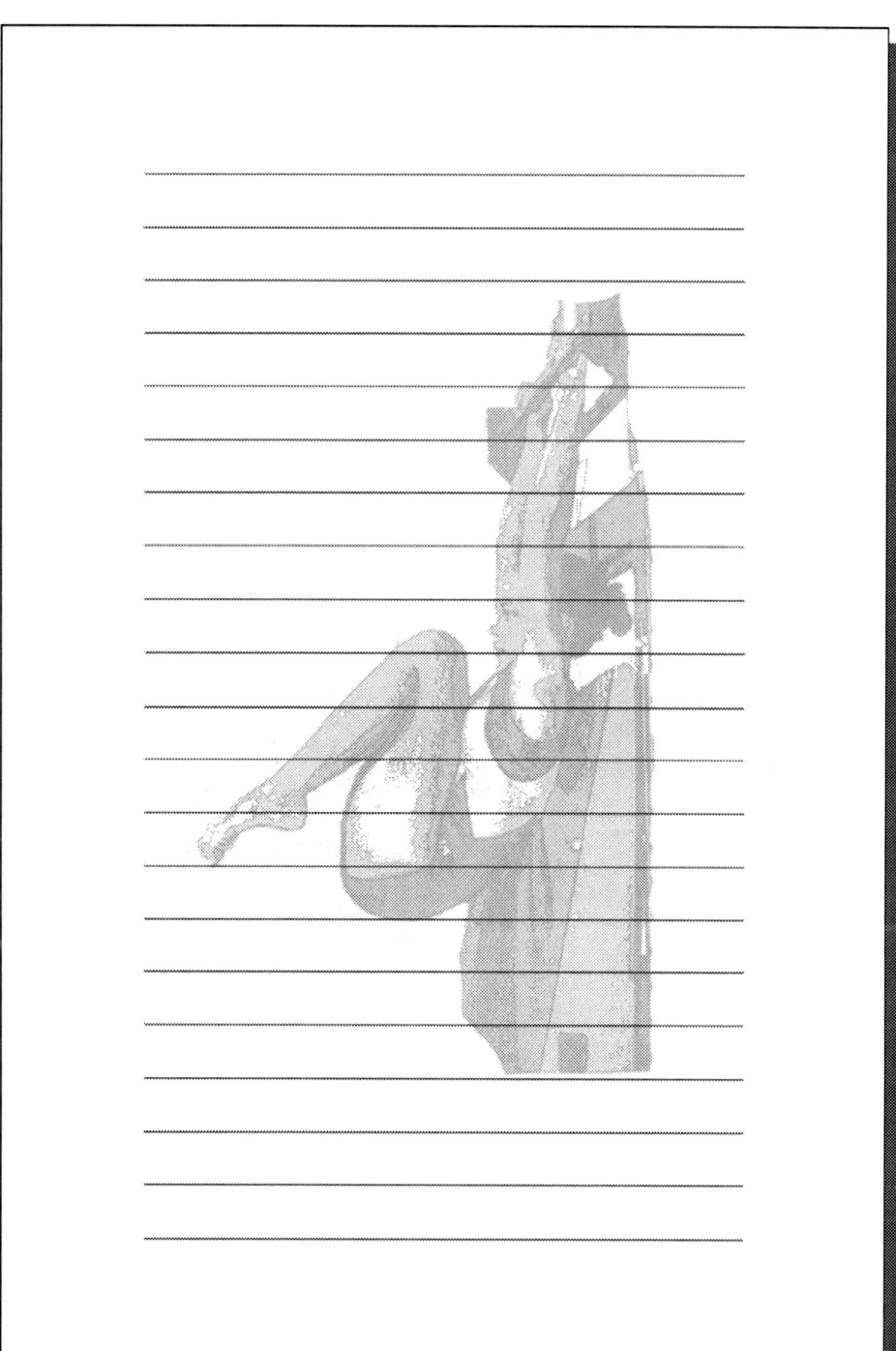

Gymnastics Journal & Meet Survival Guide

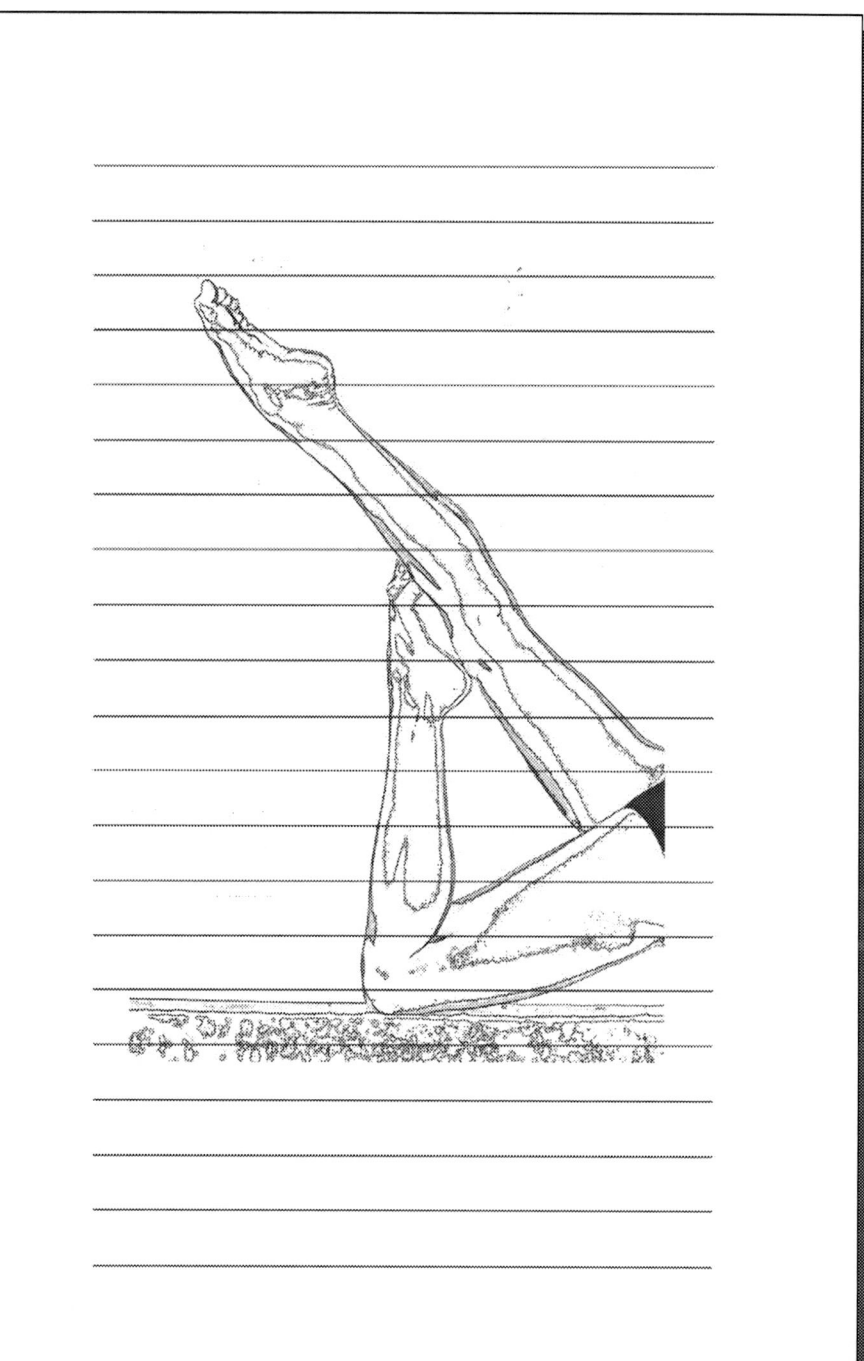

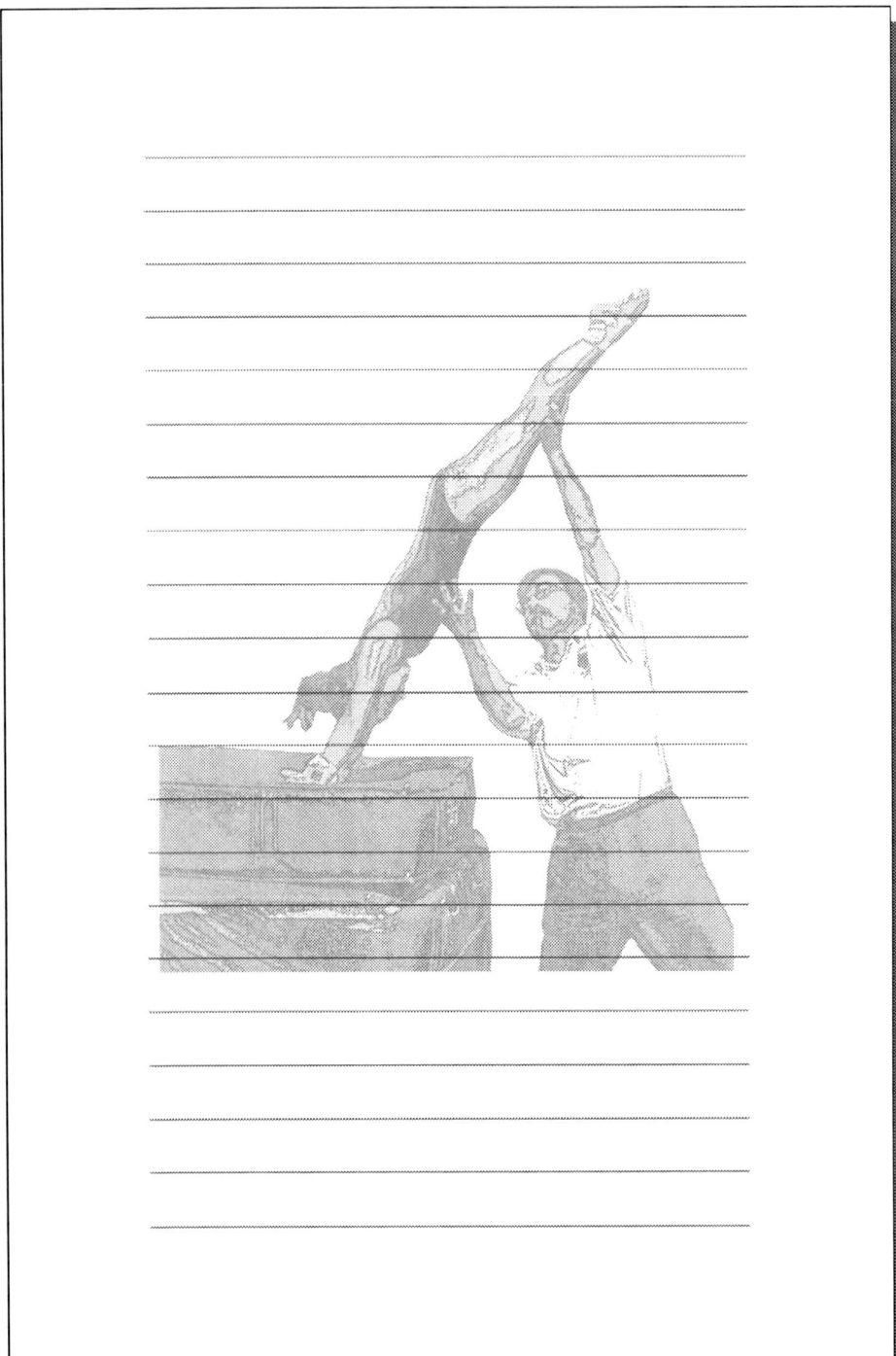

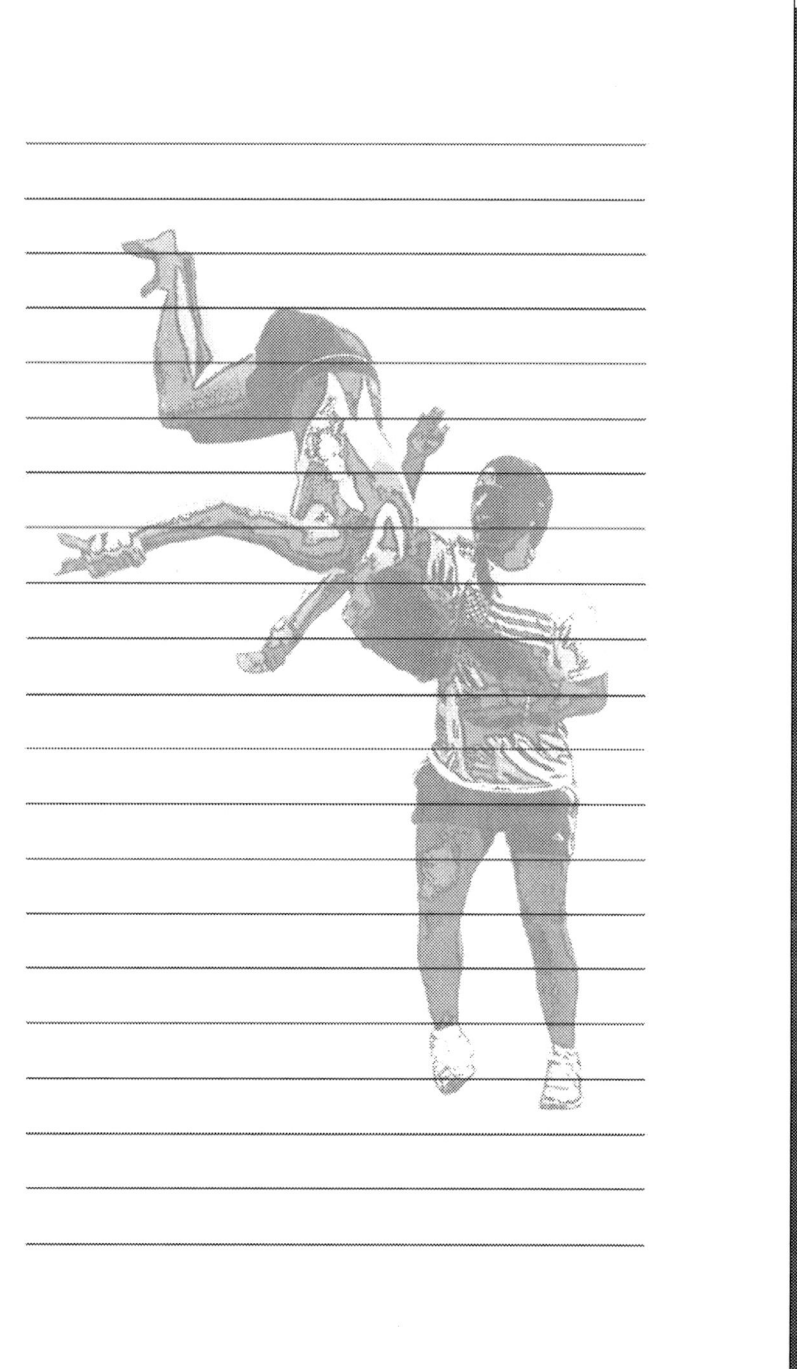

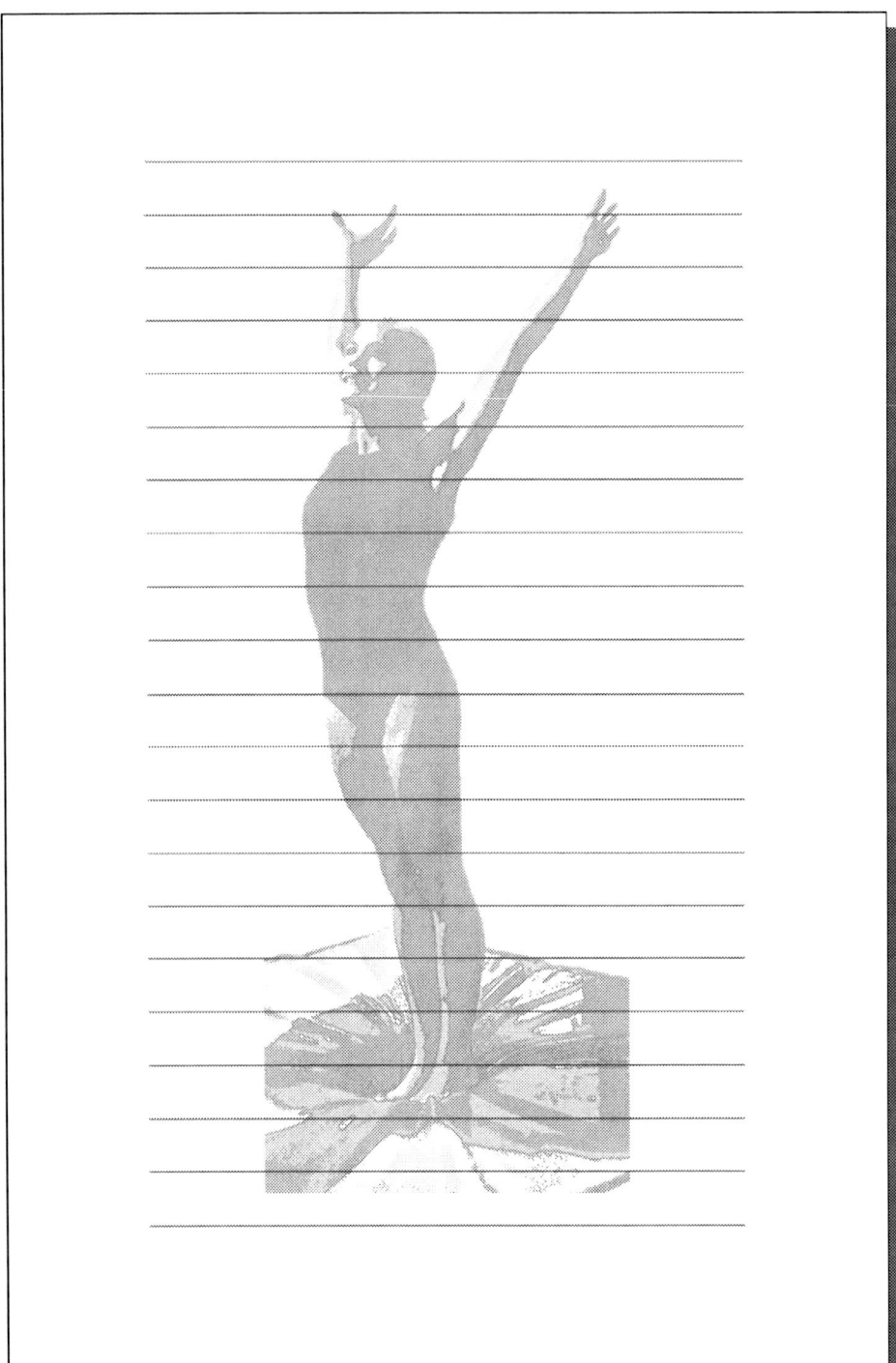

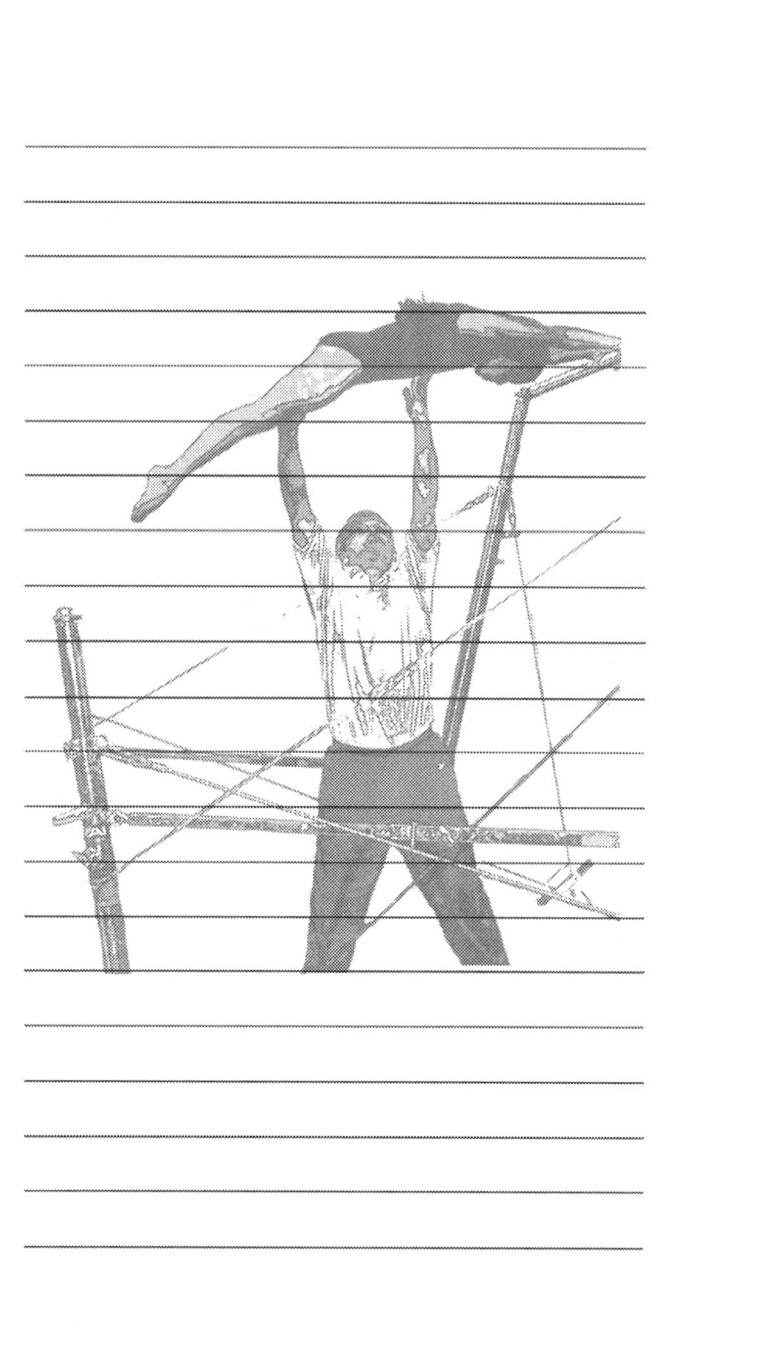

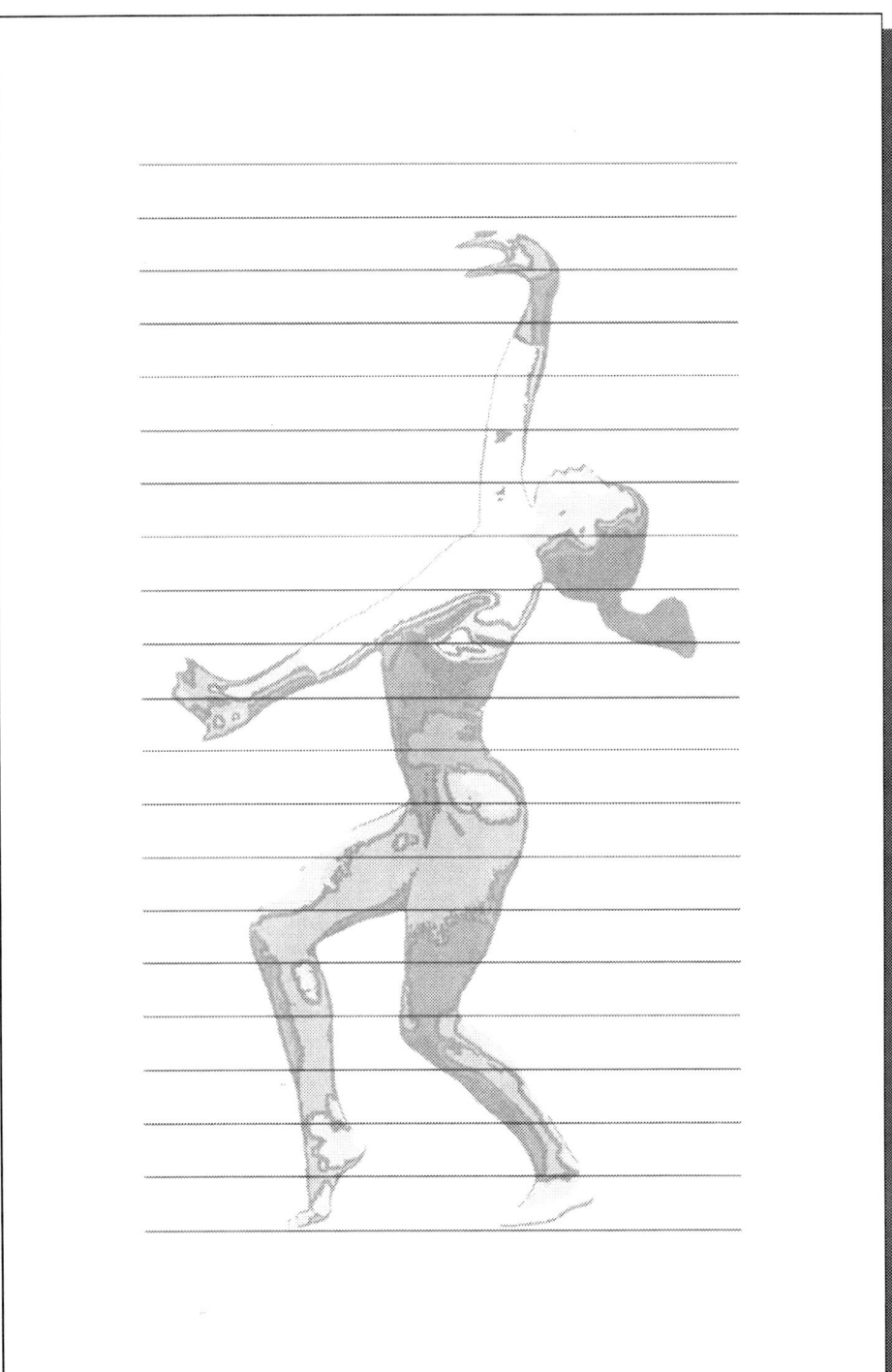

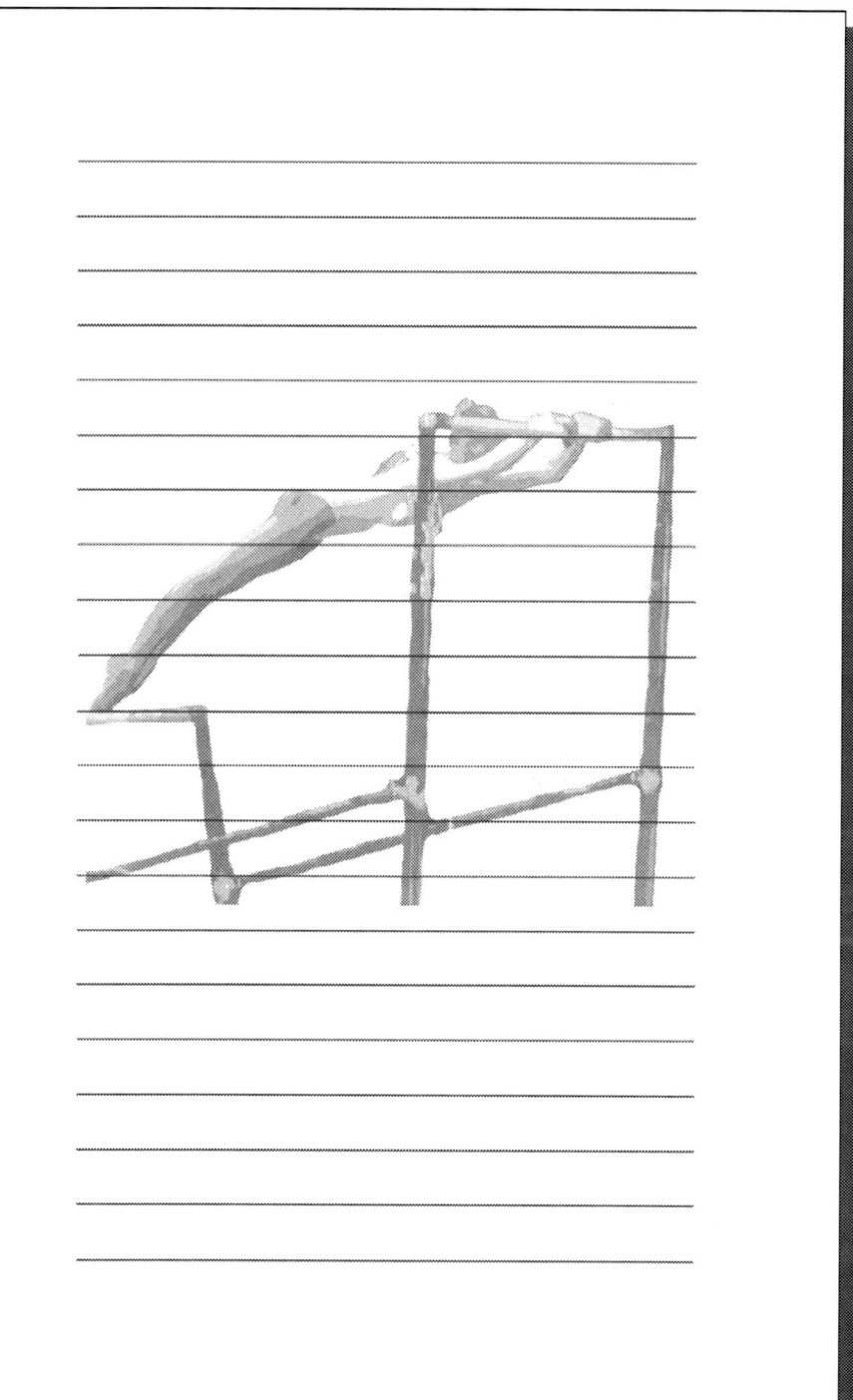

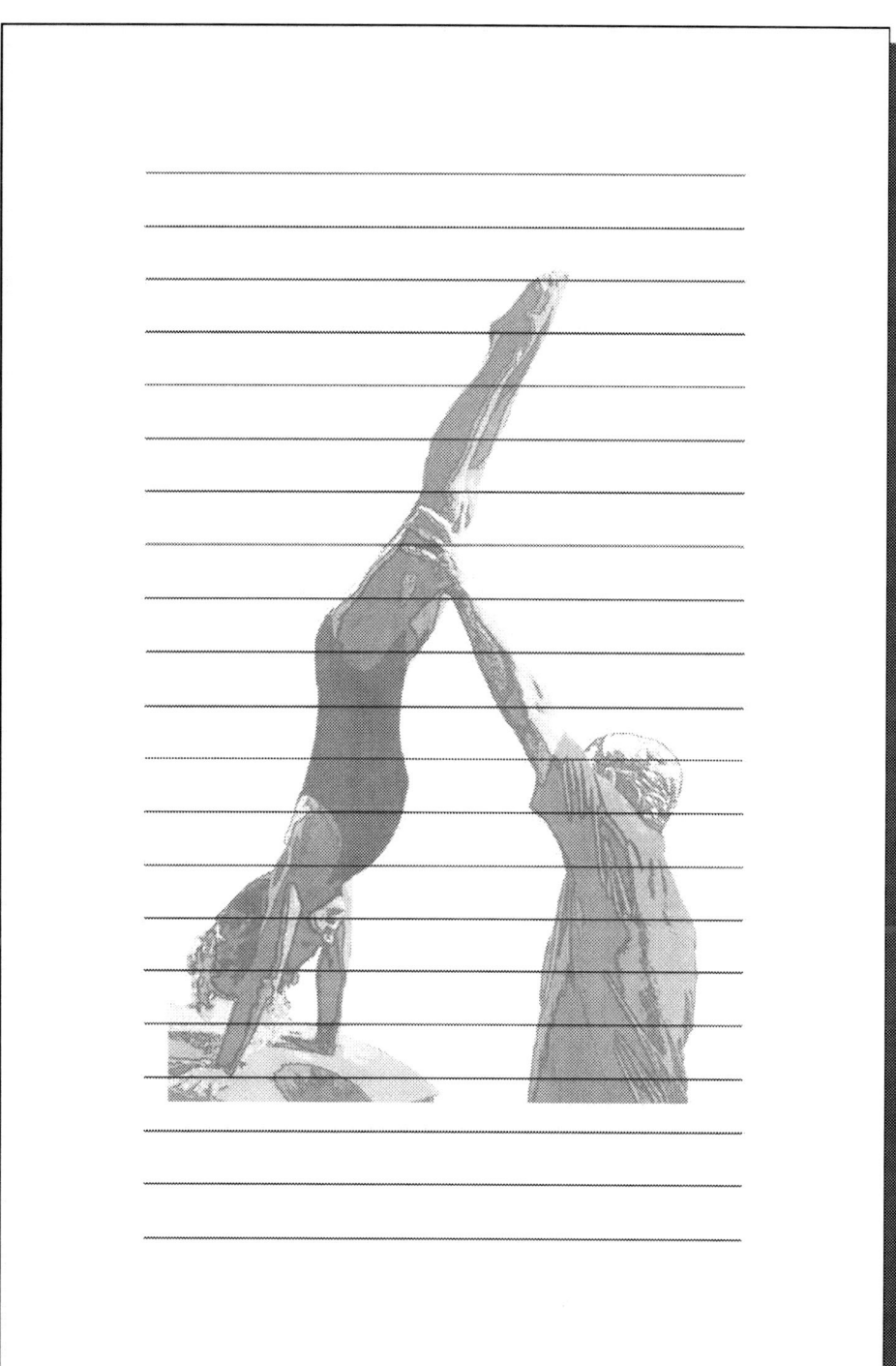

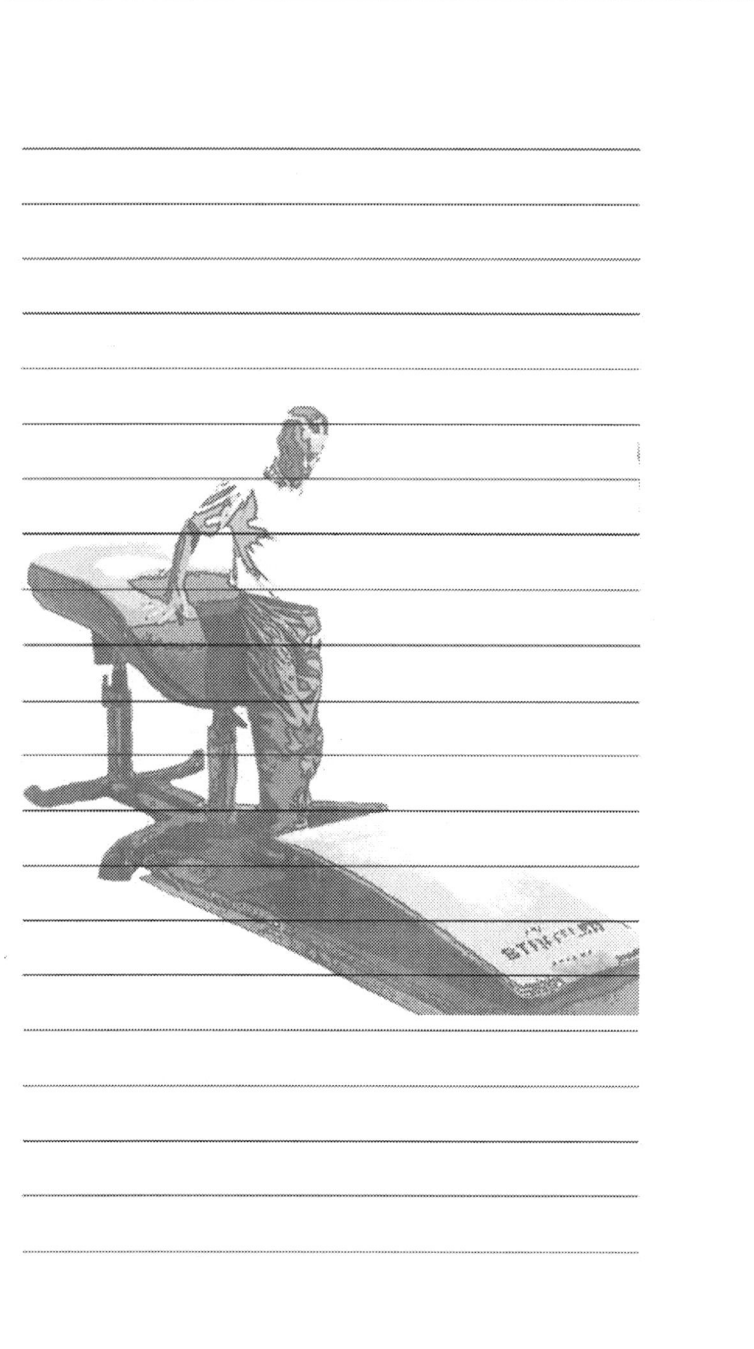

Gymnastics Journal & Meet Survival Guide

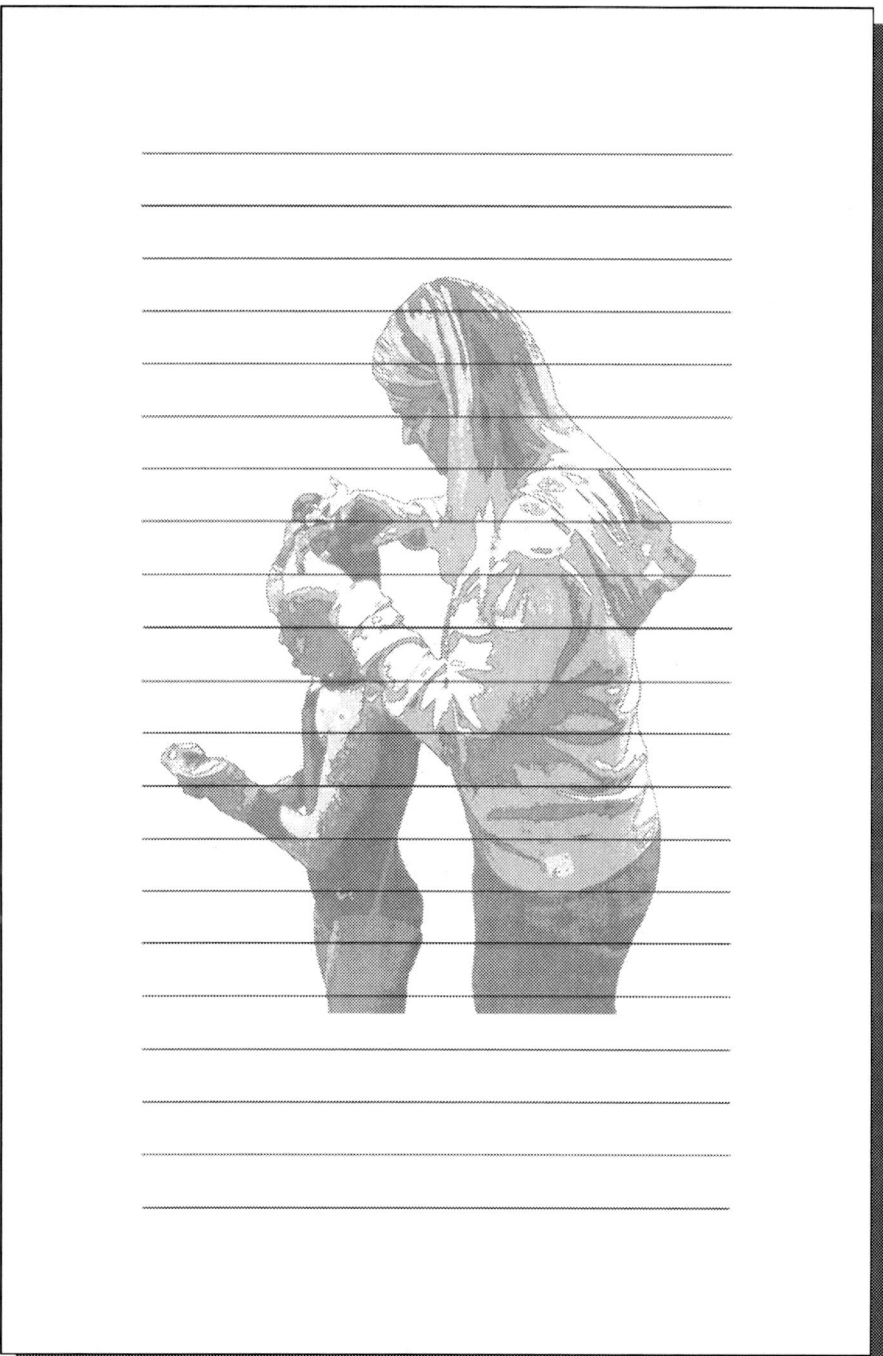

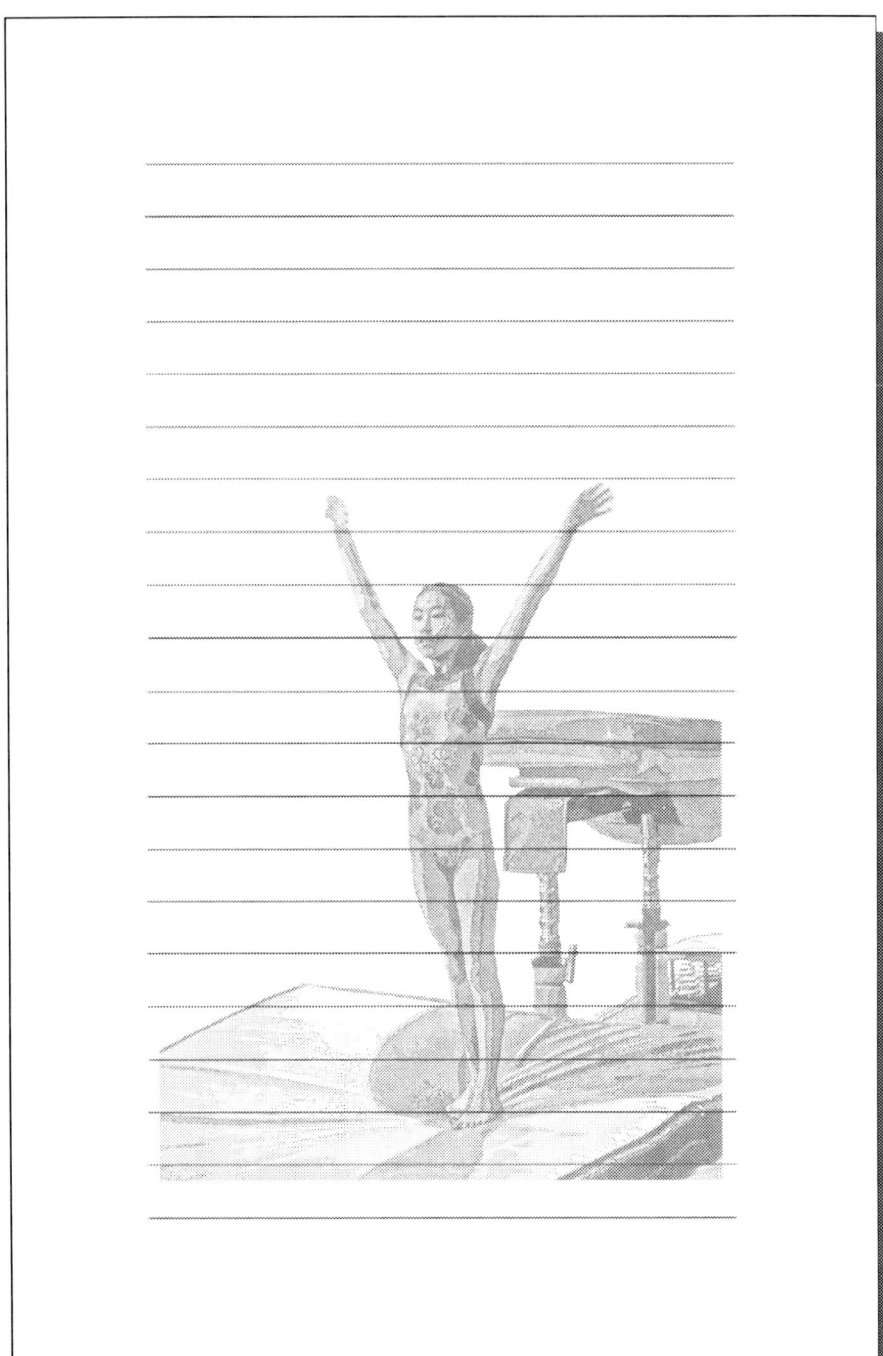

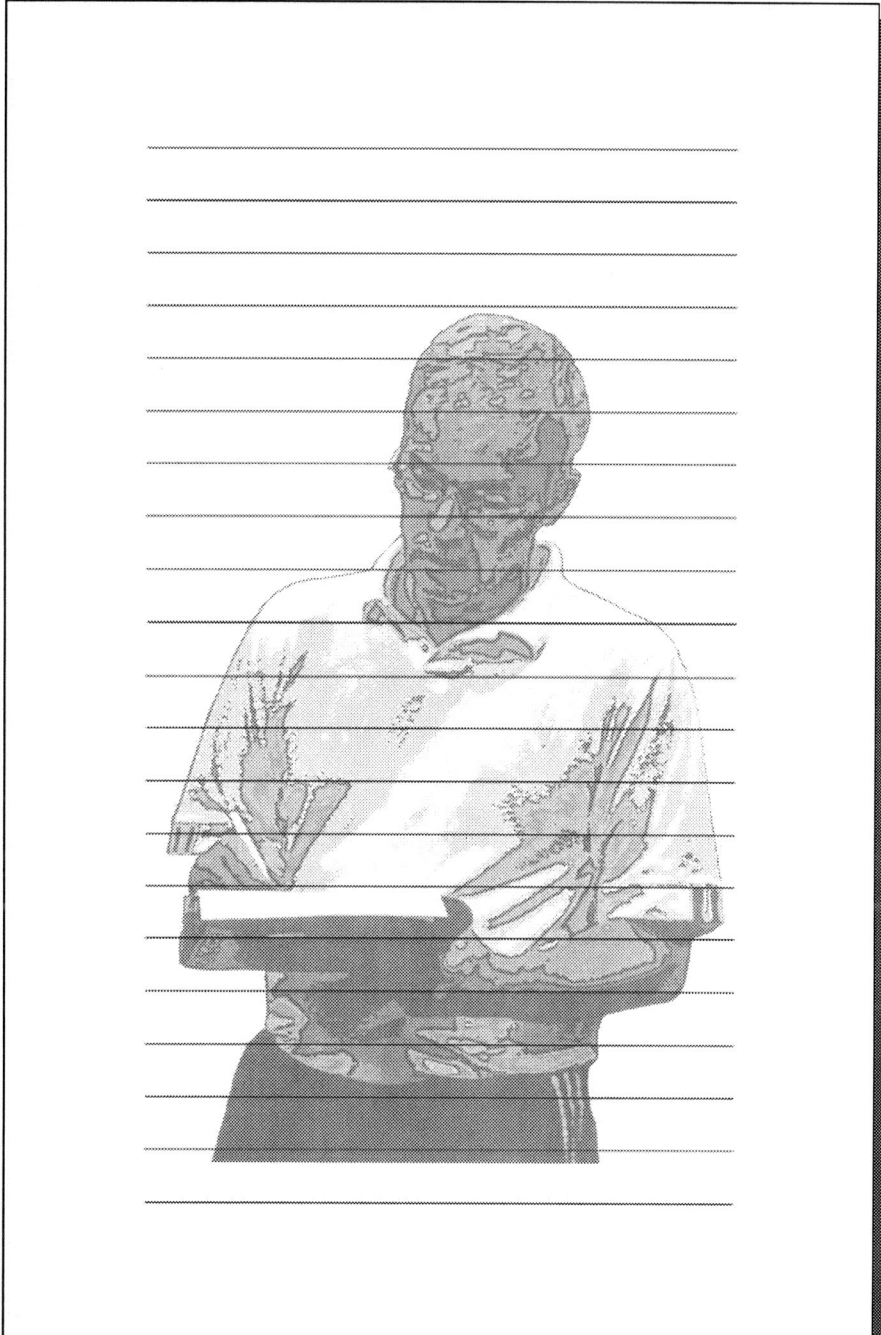

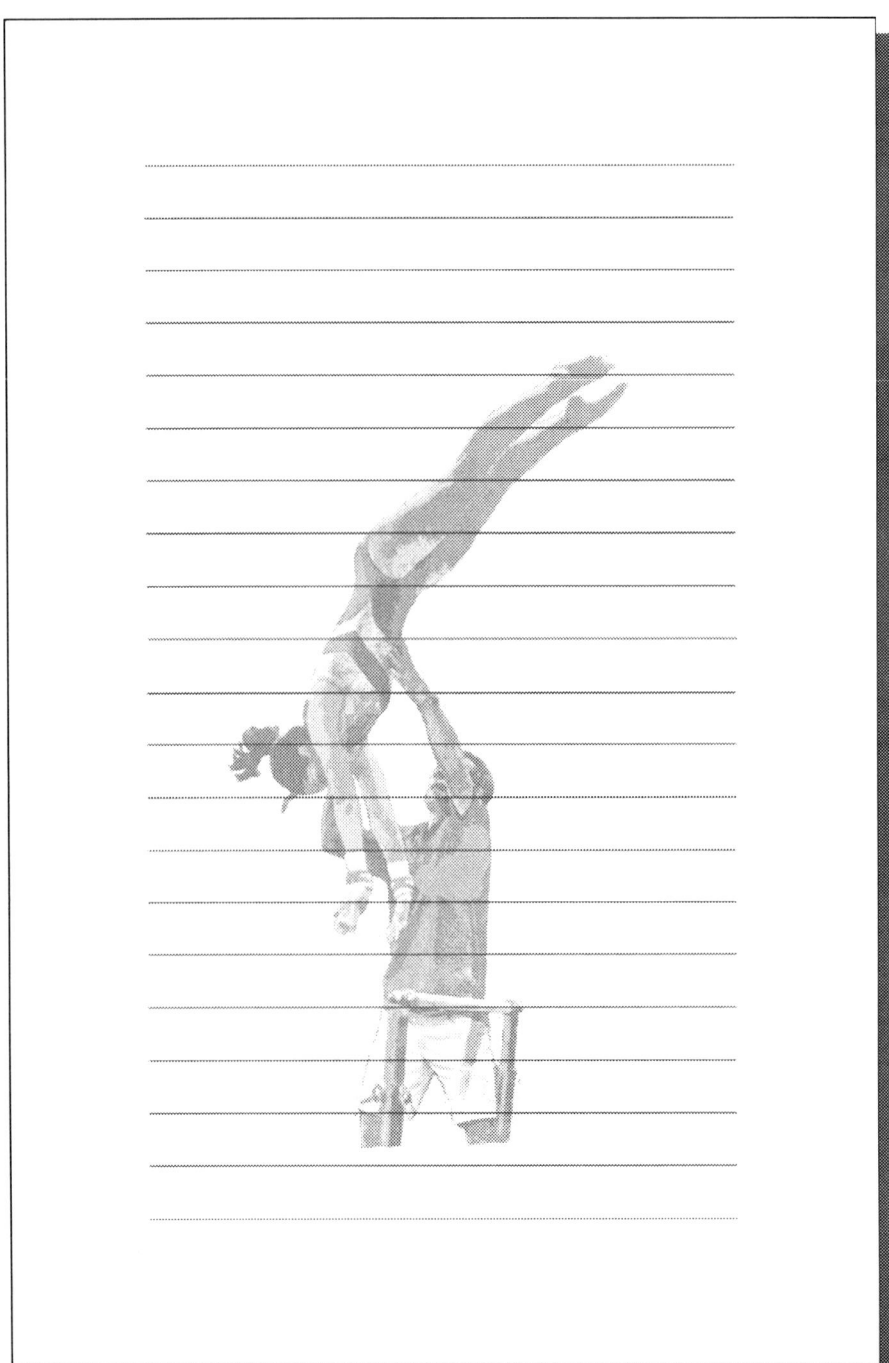

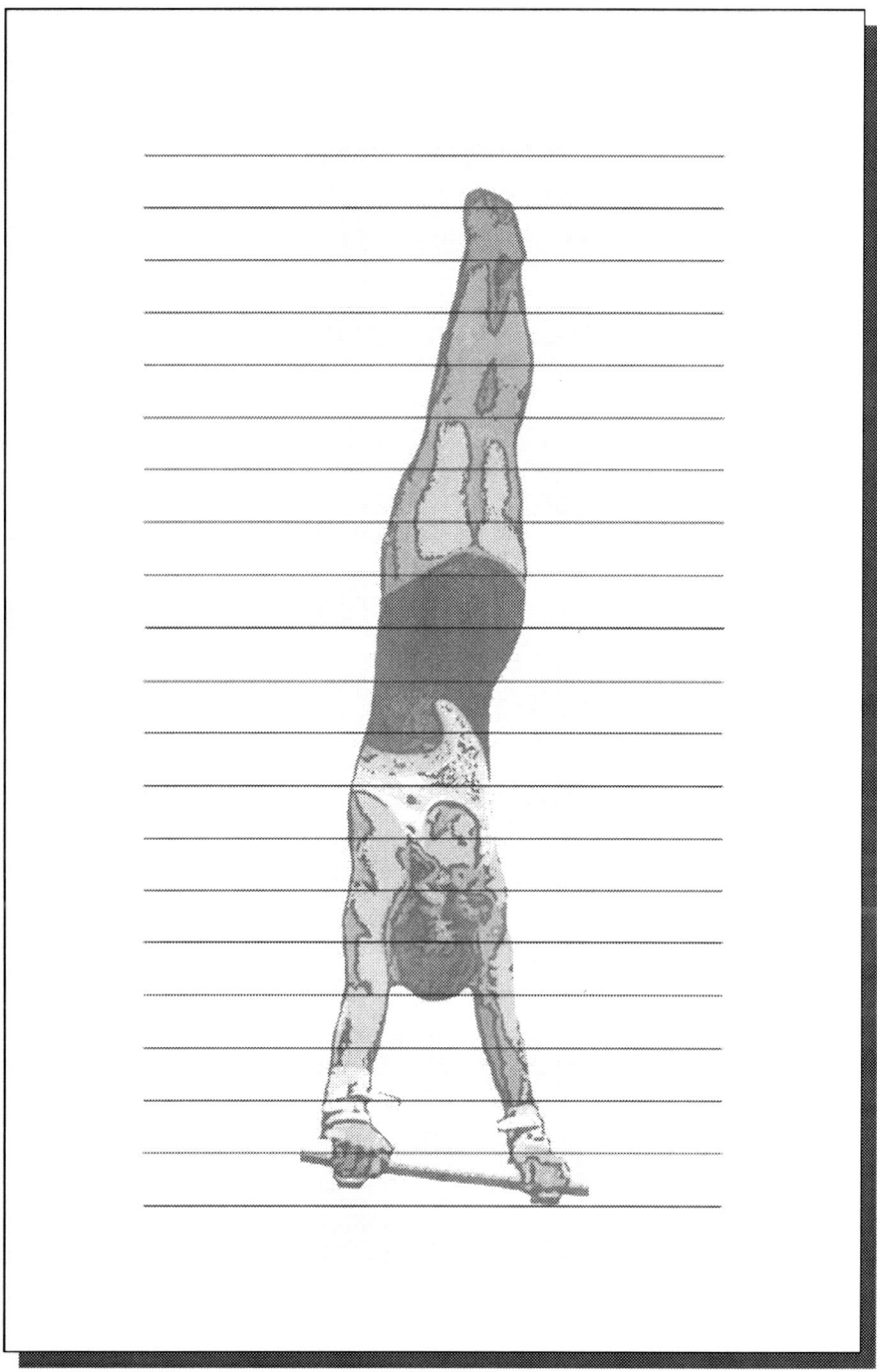

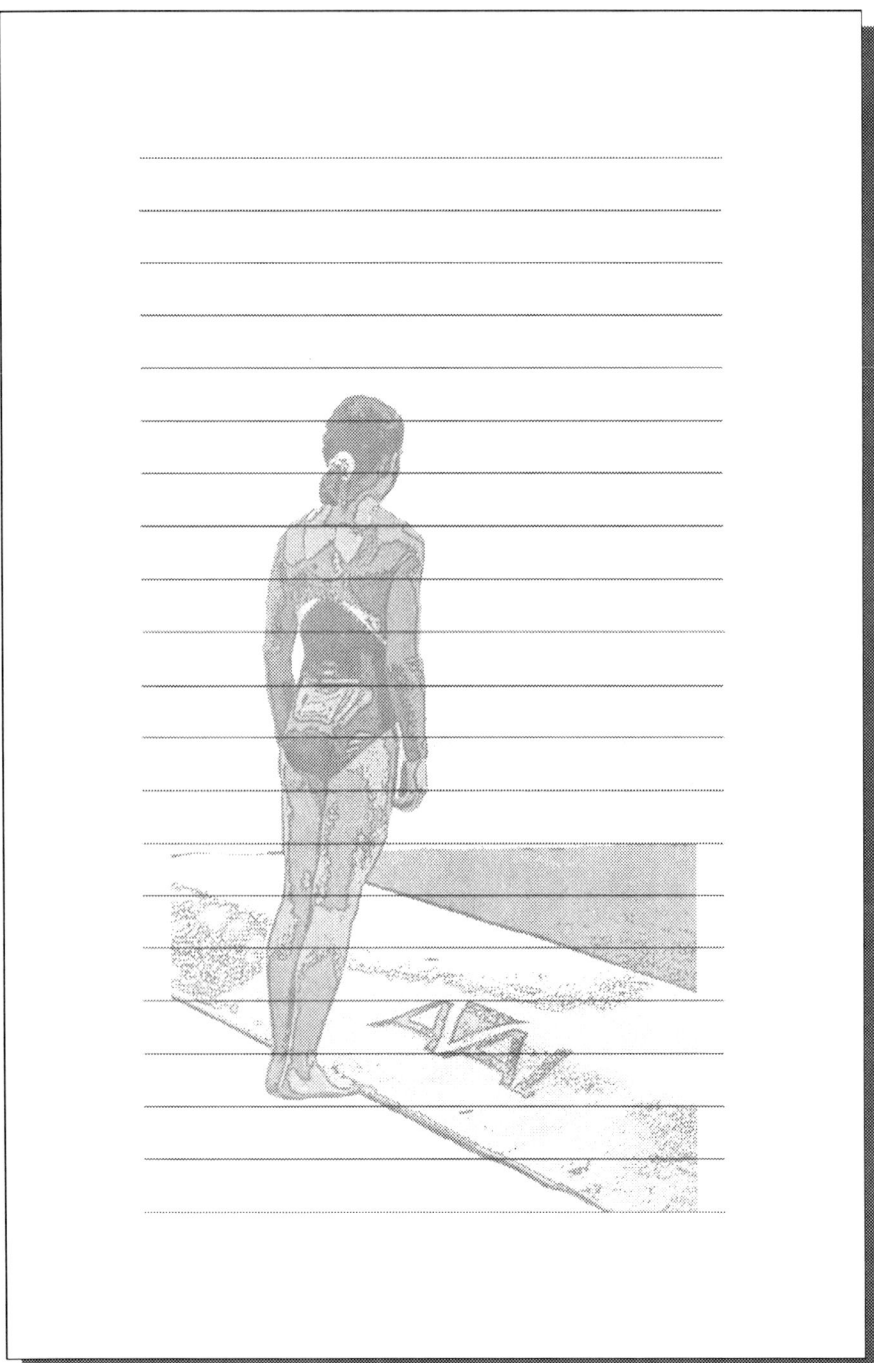

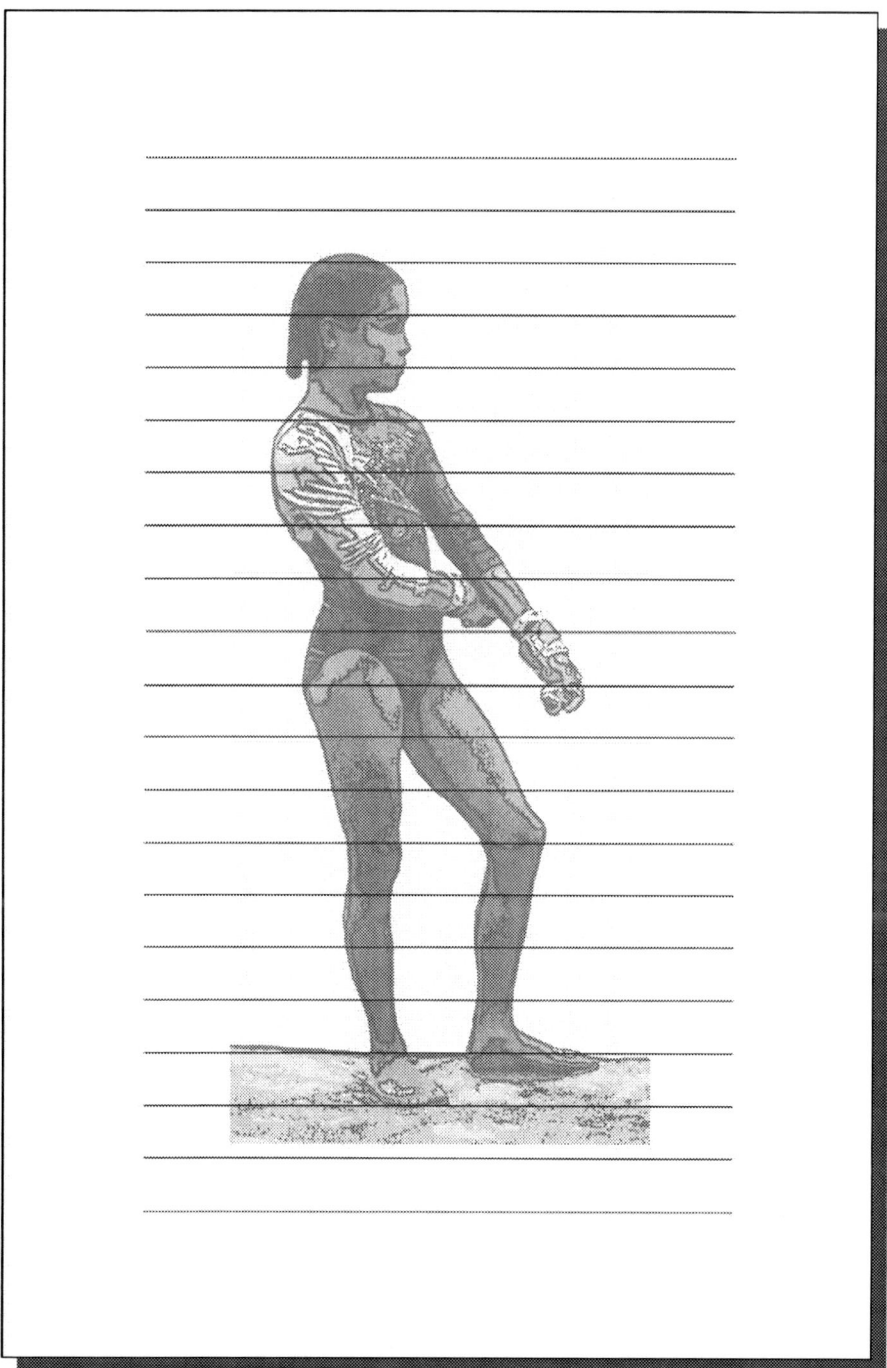

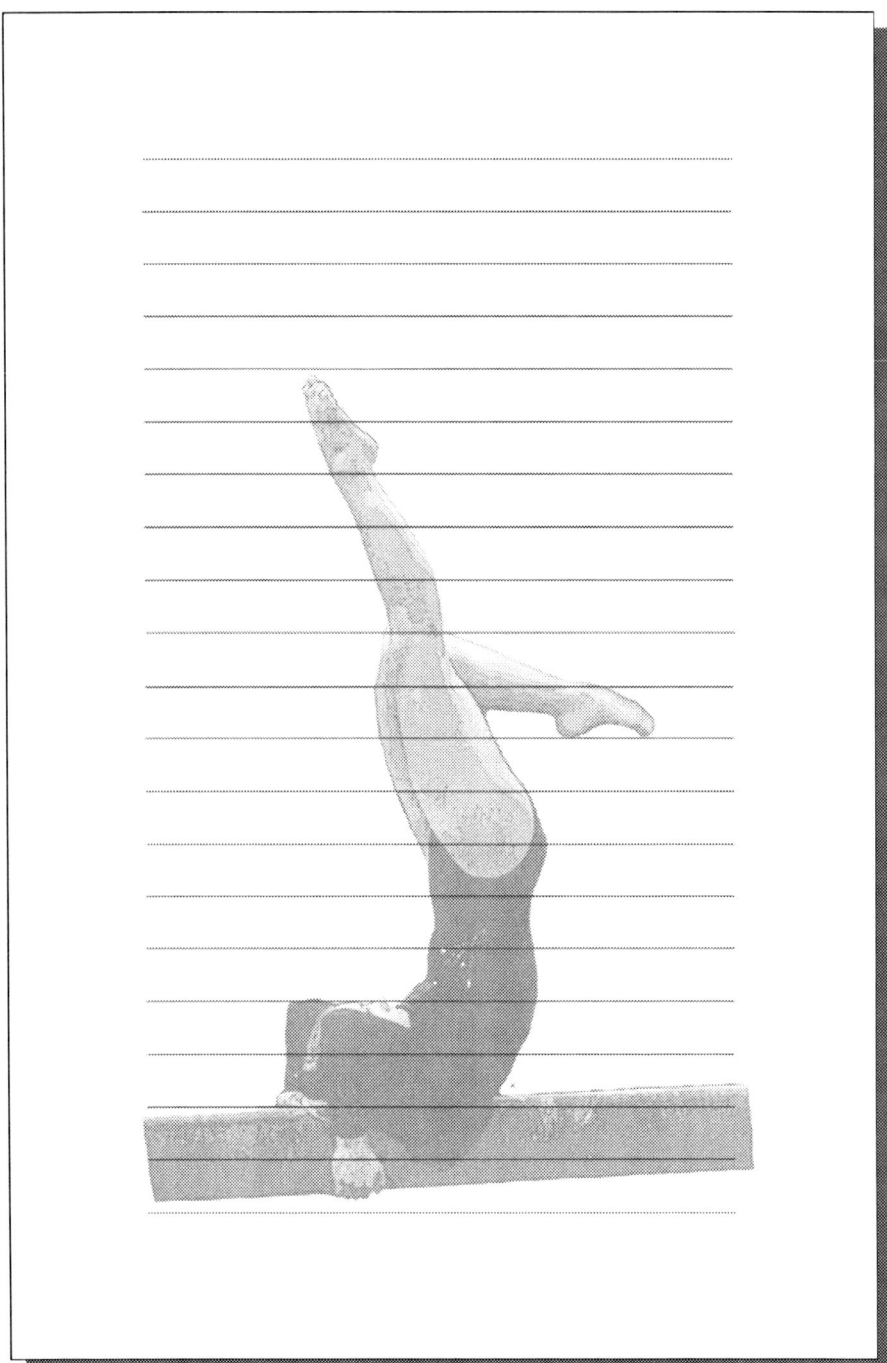

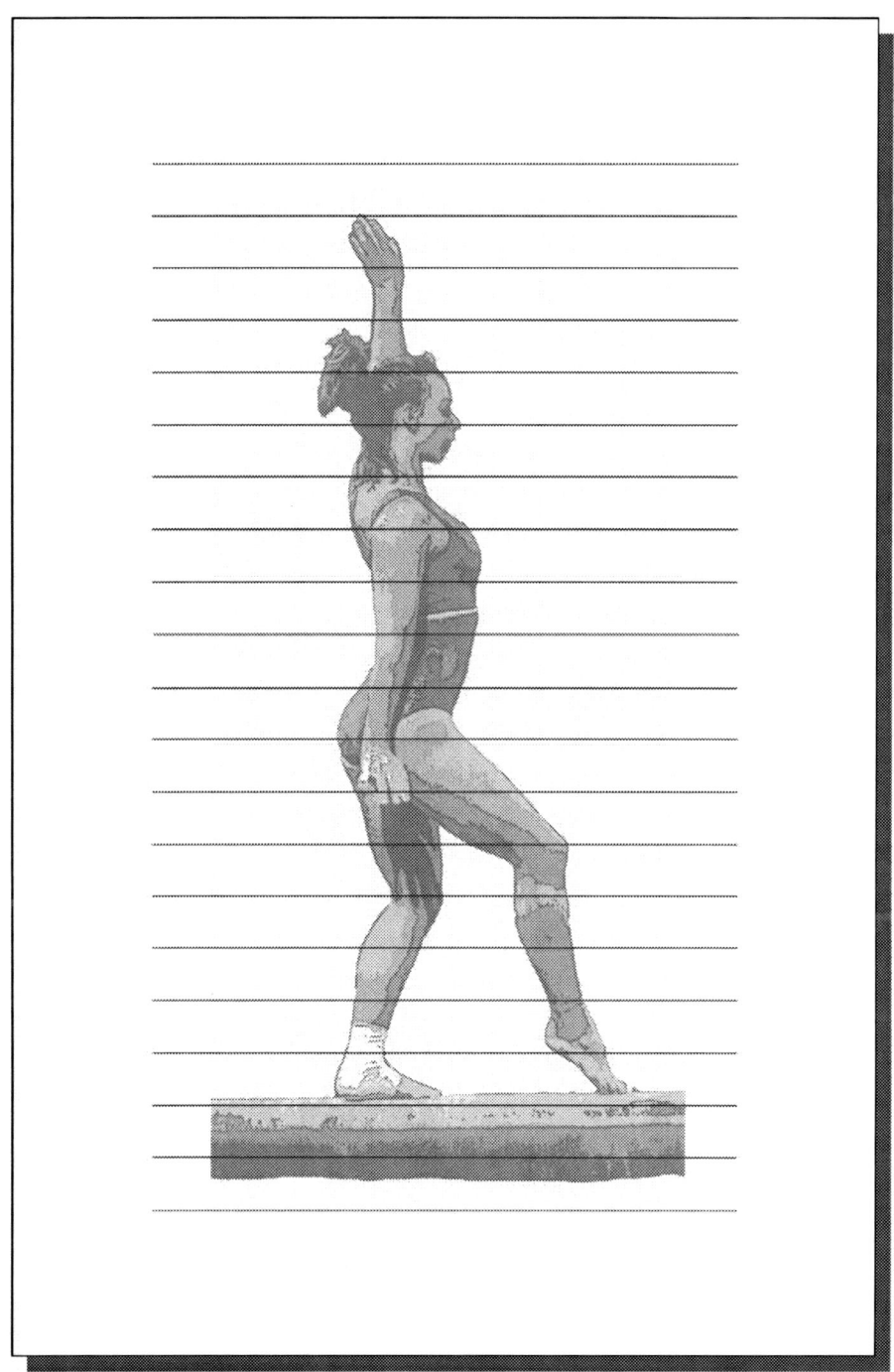

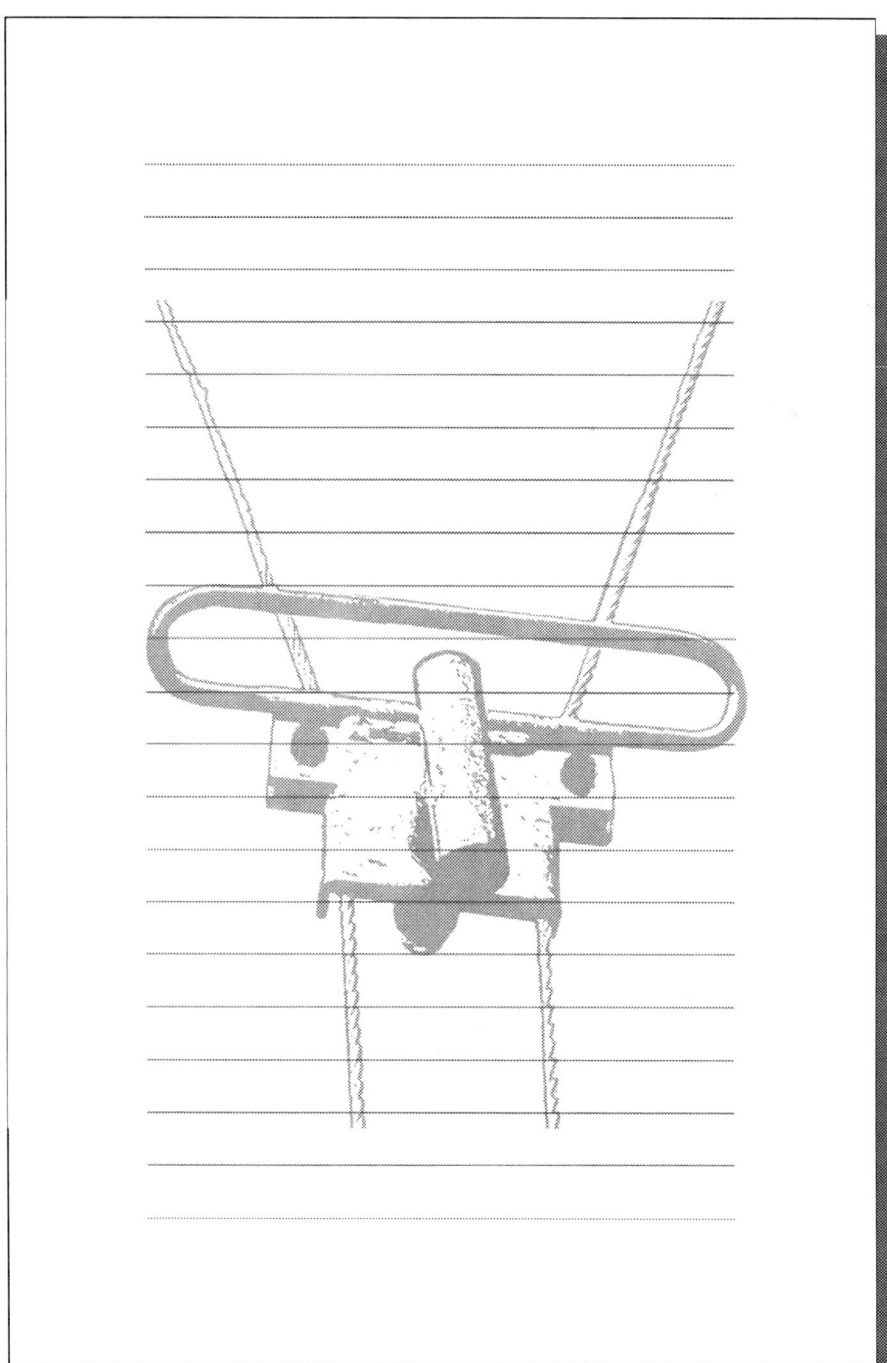

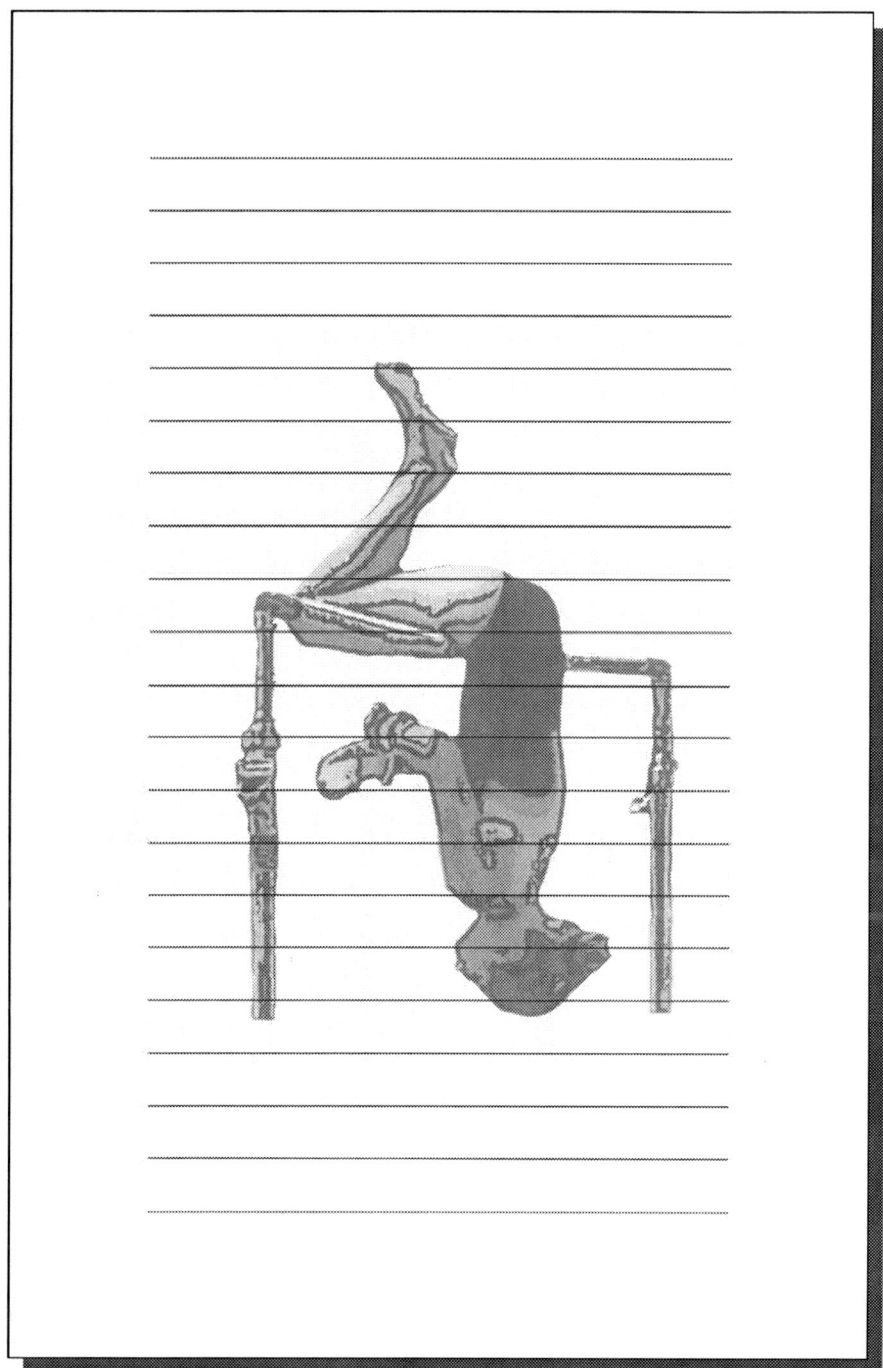

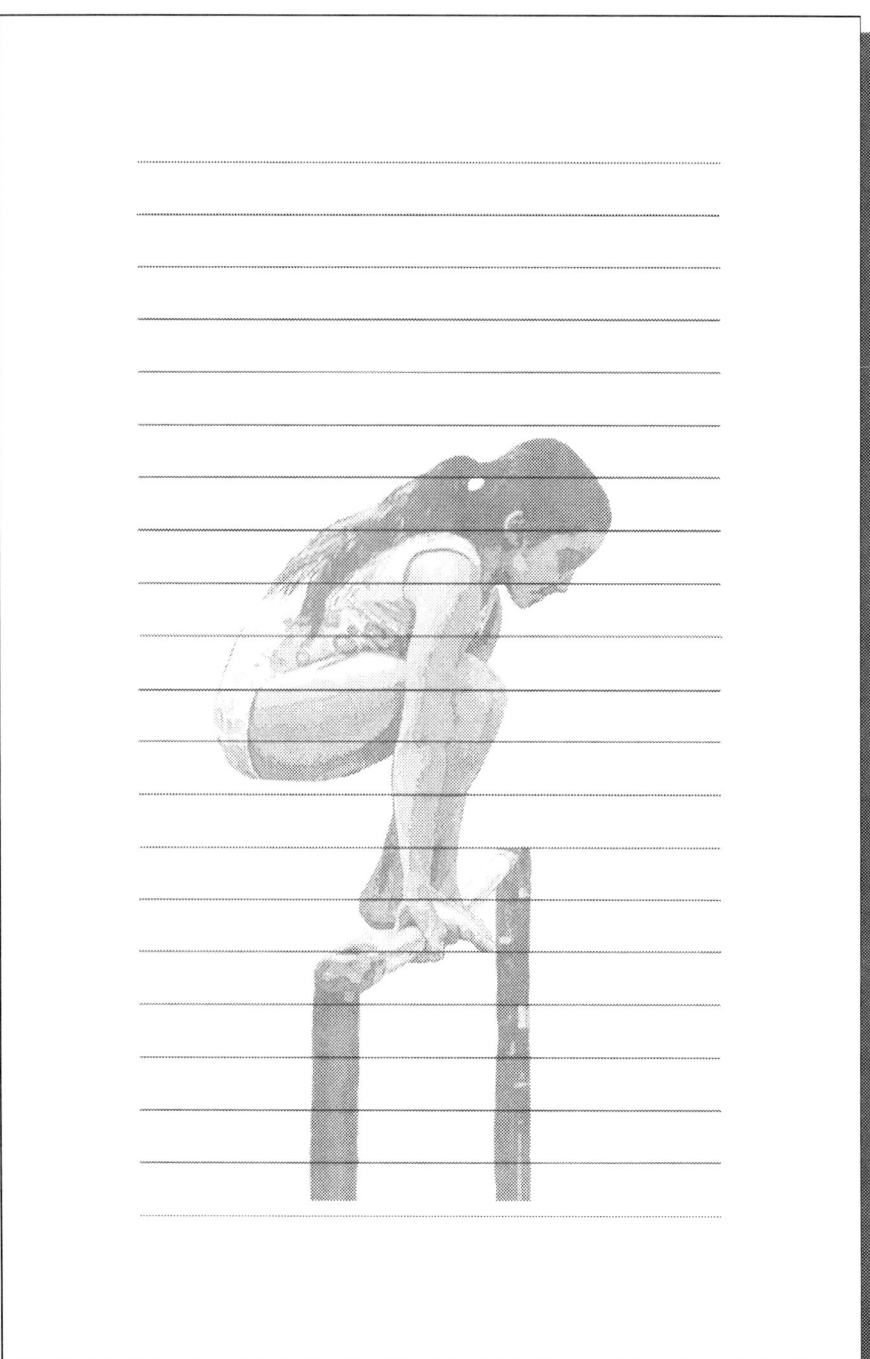

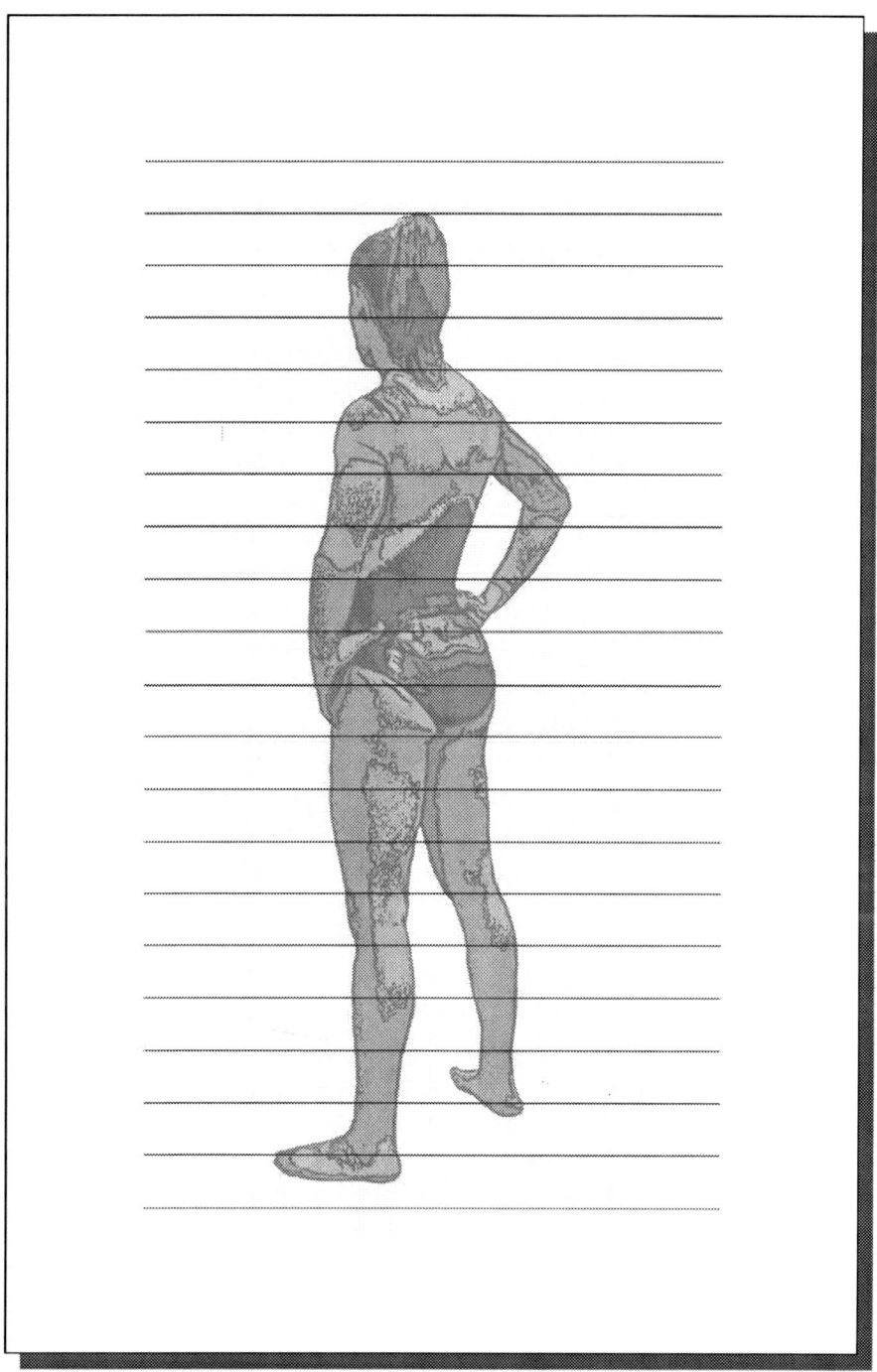

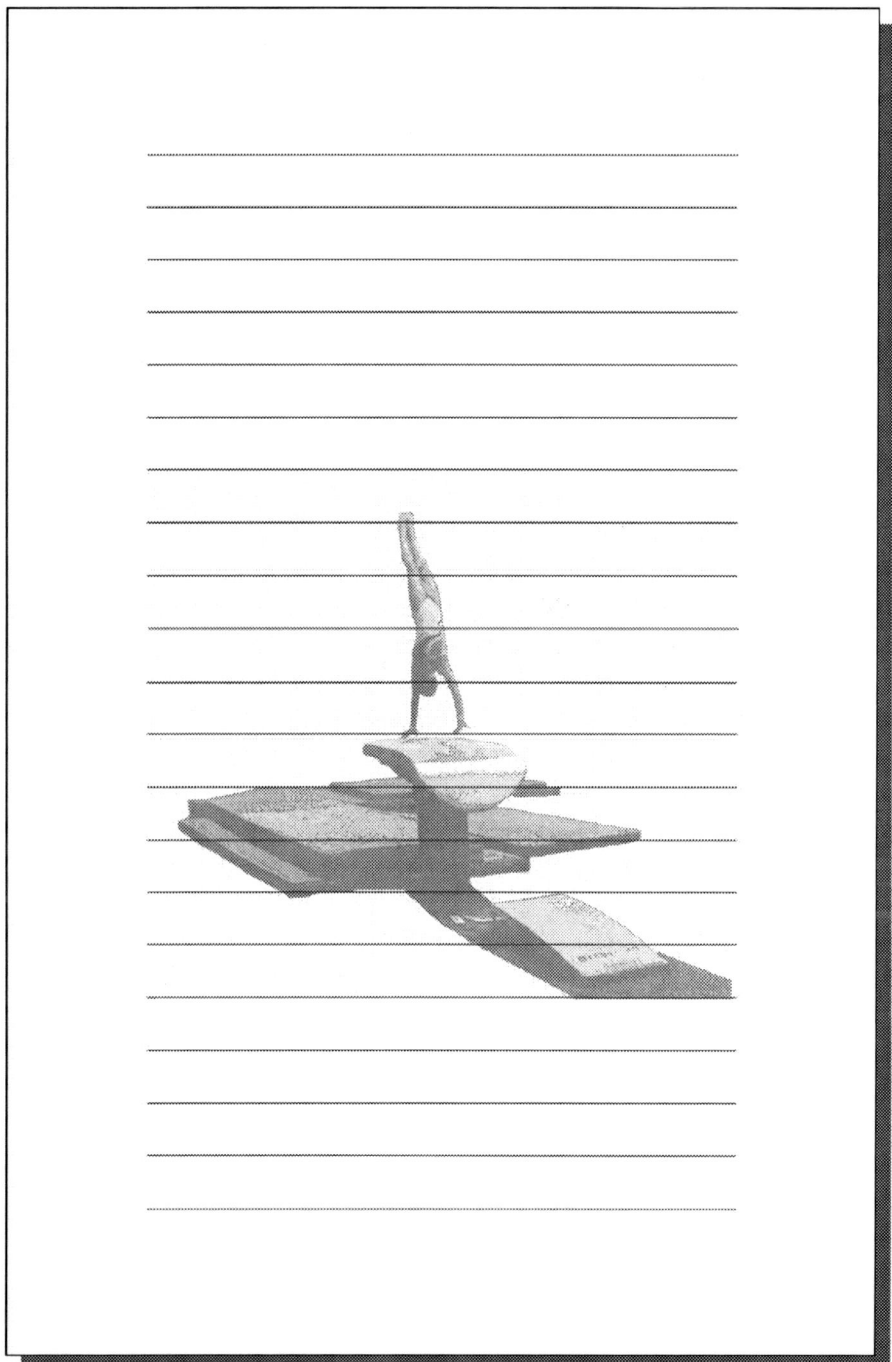

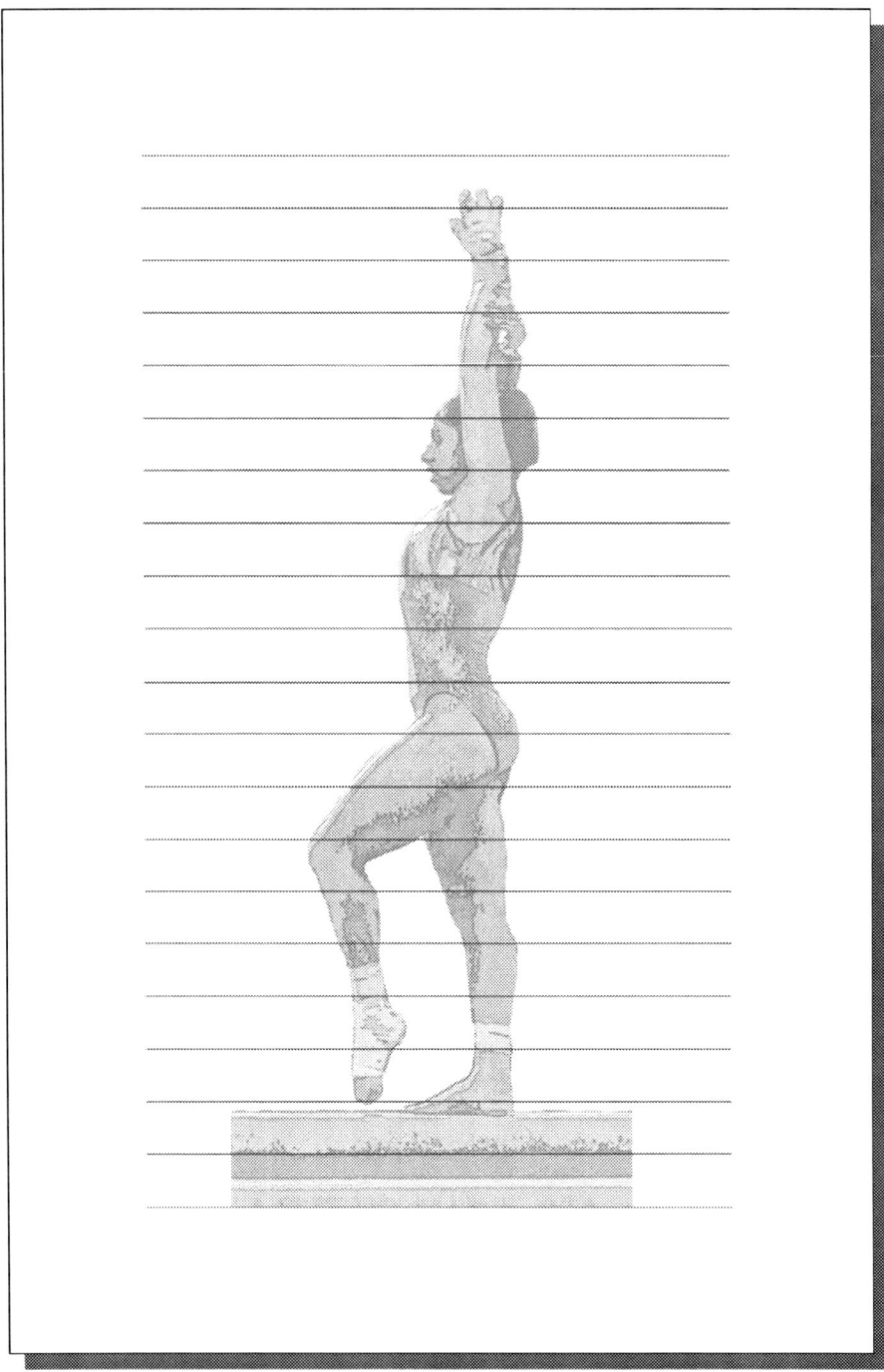

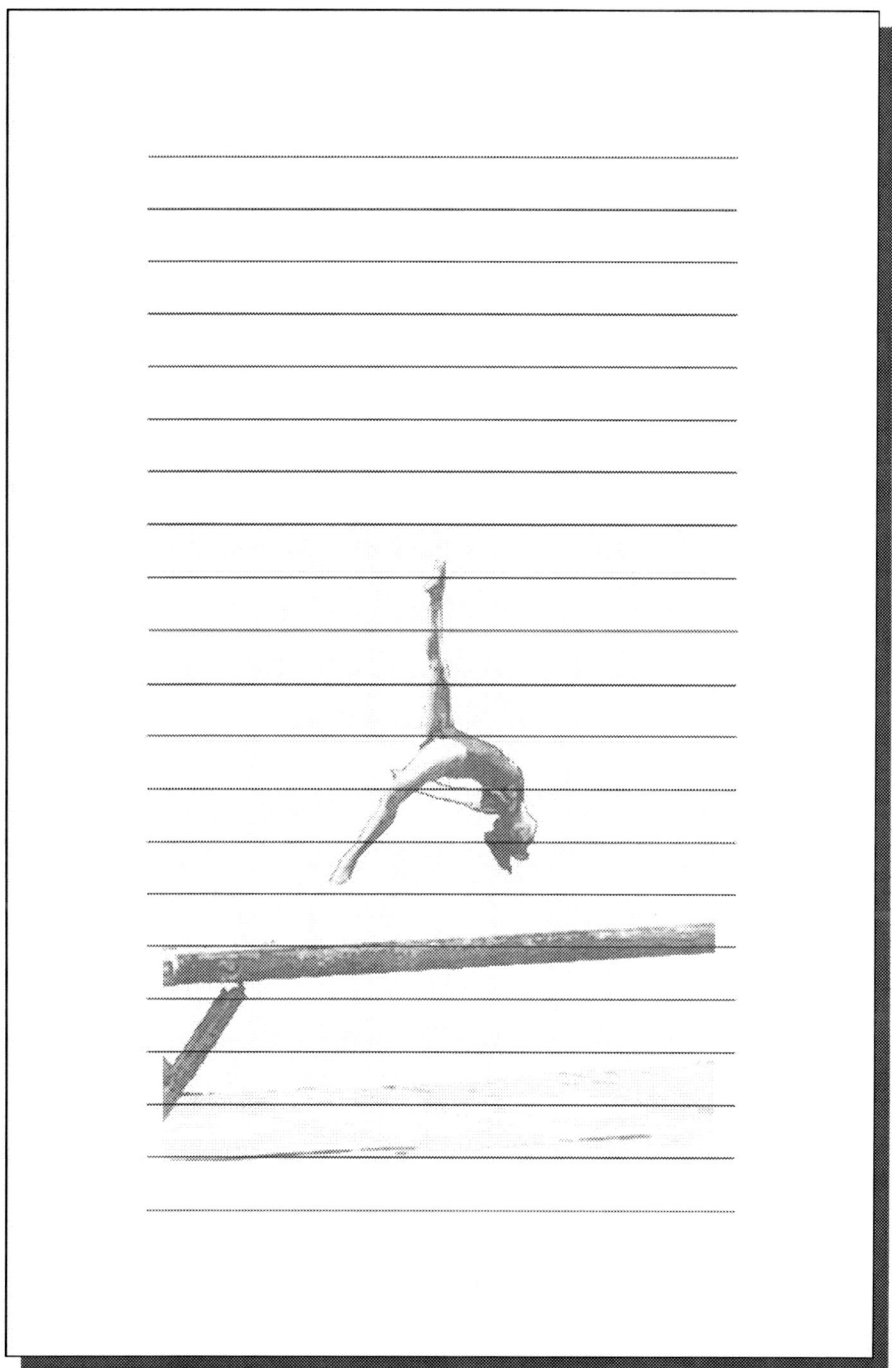

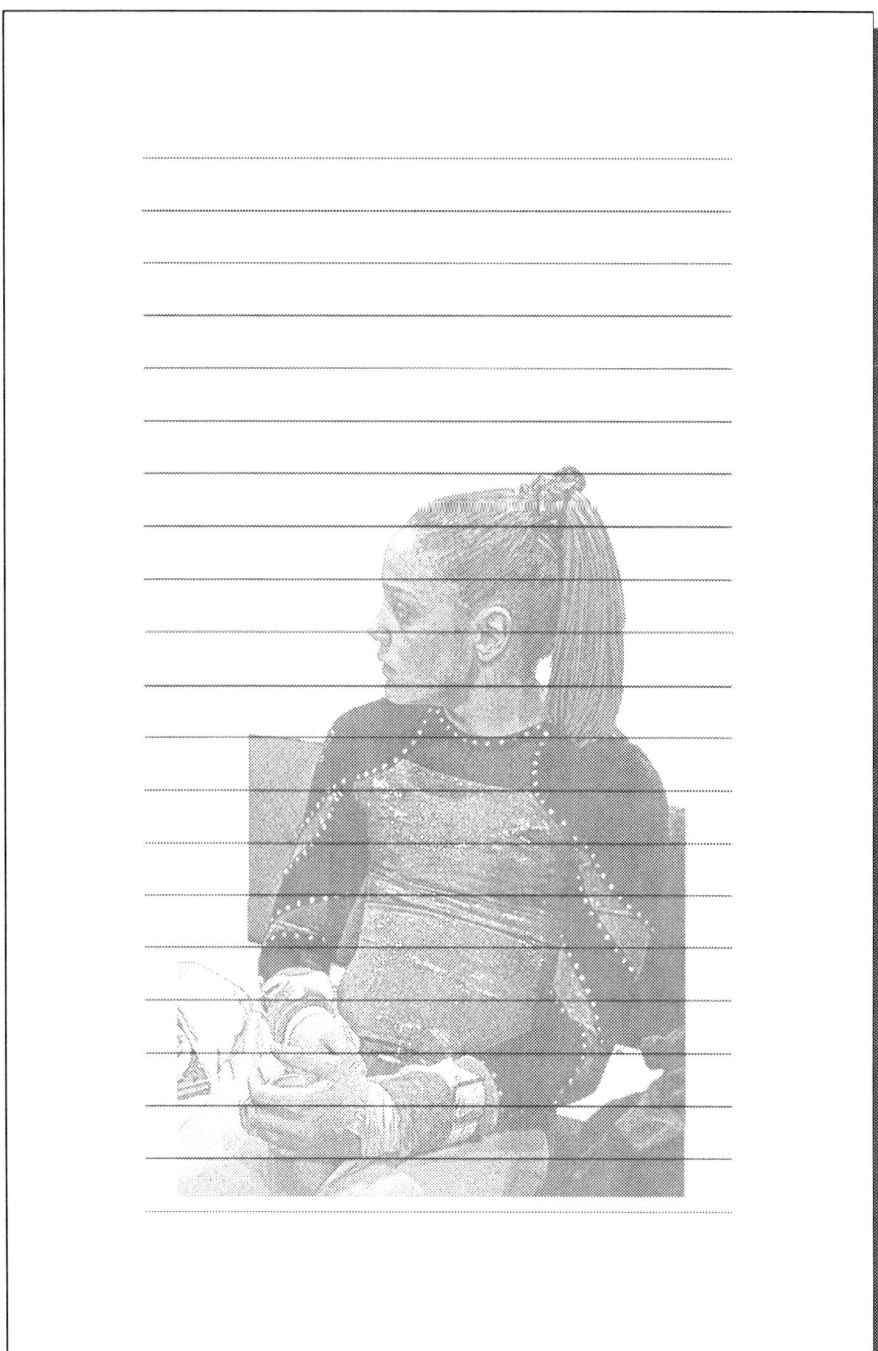

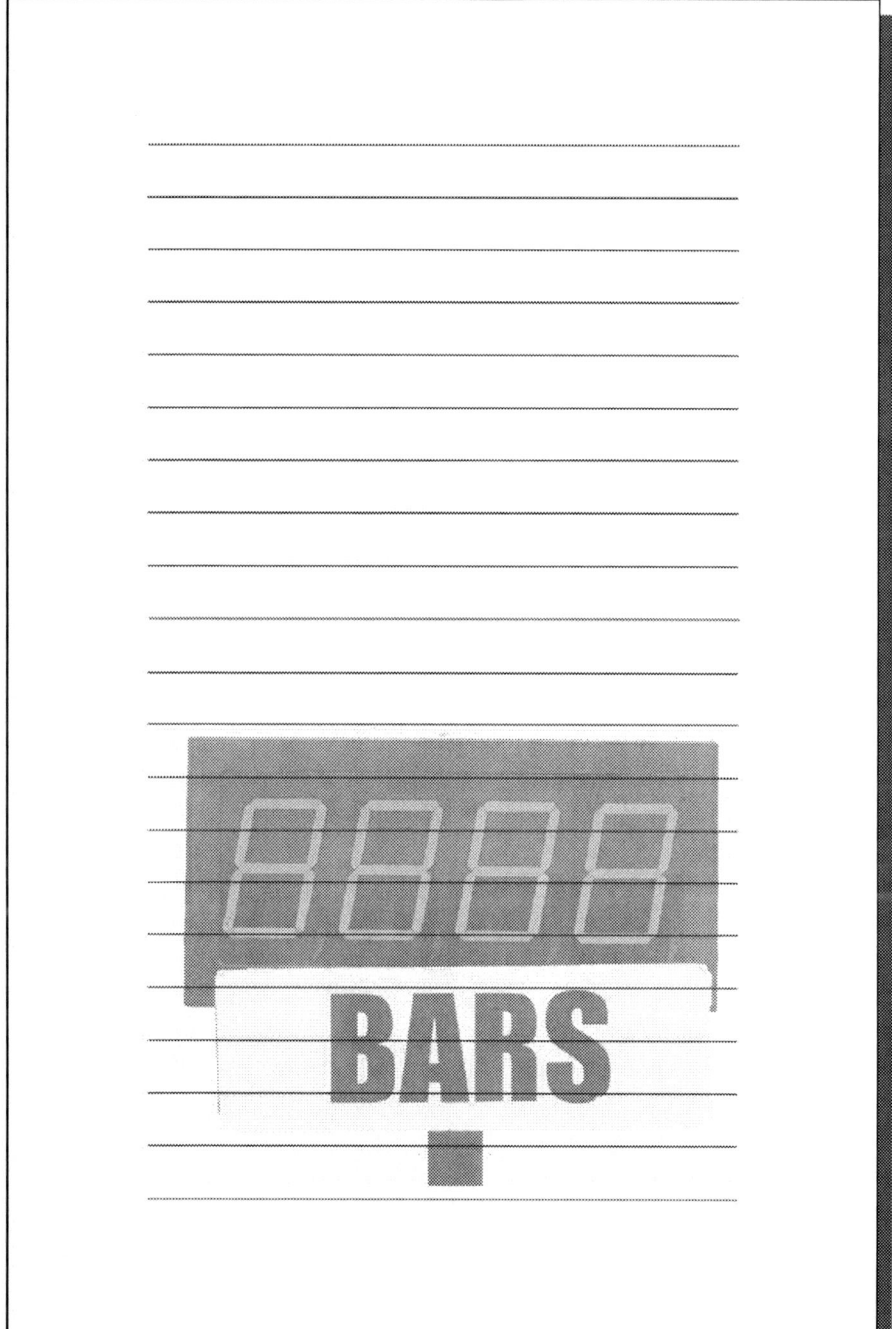

Gymnastics Journal & Meet Survival Guide

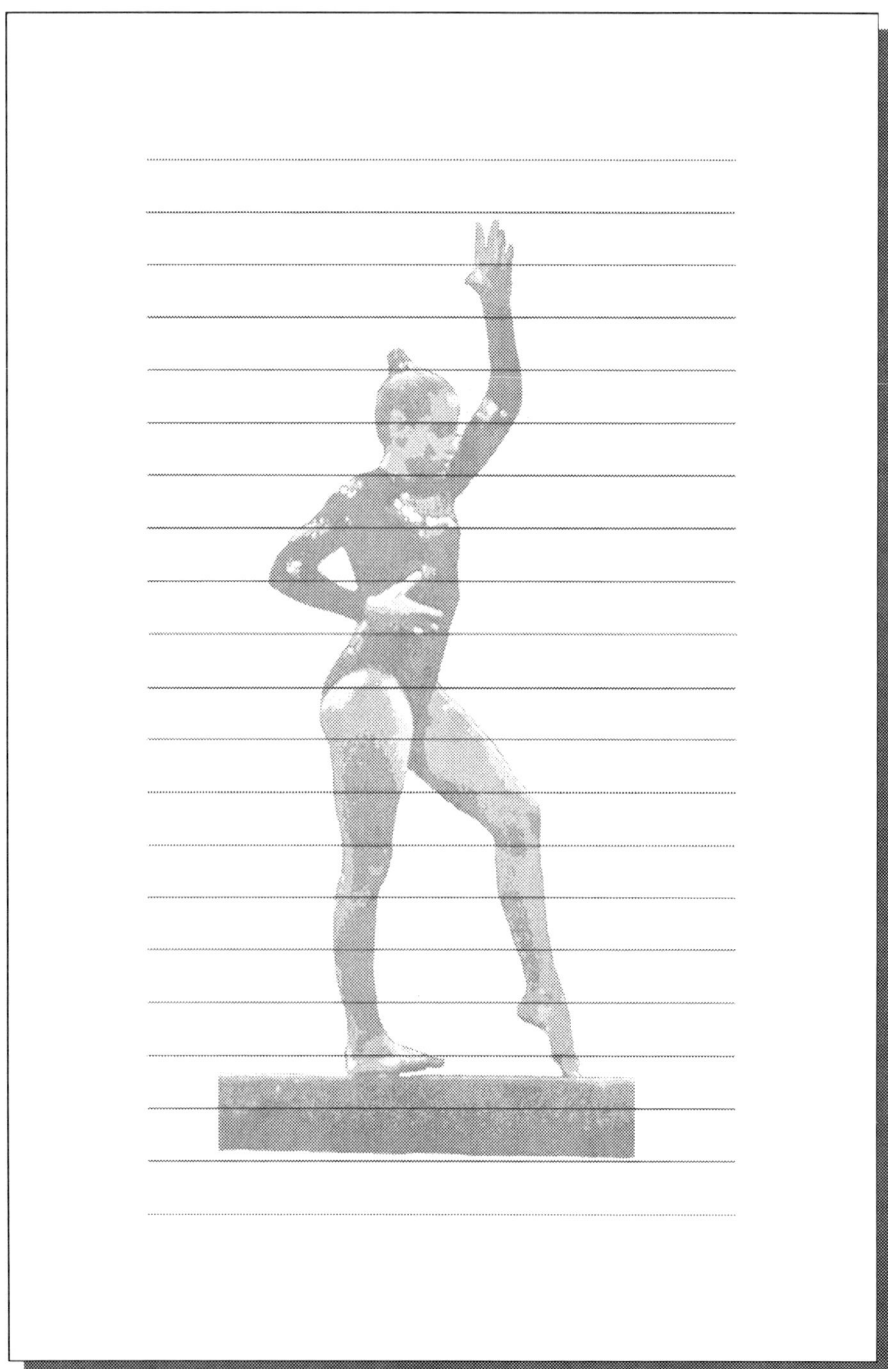

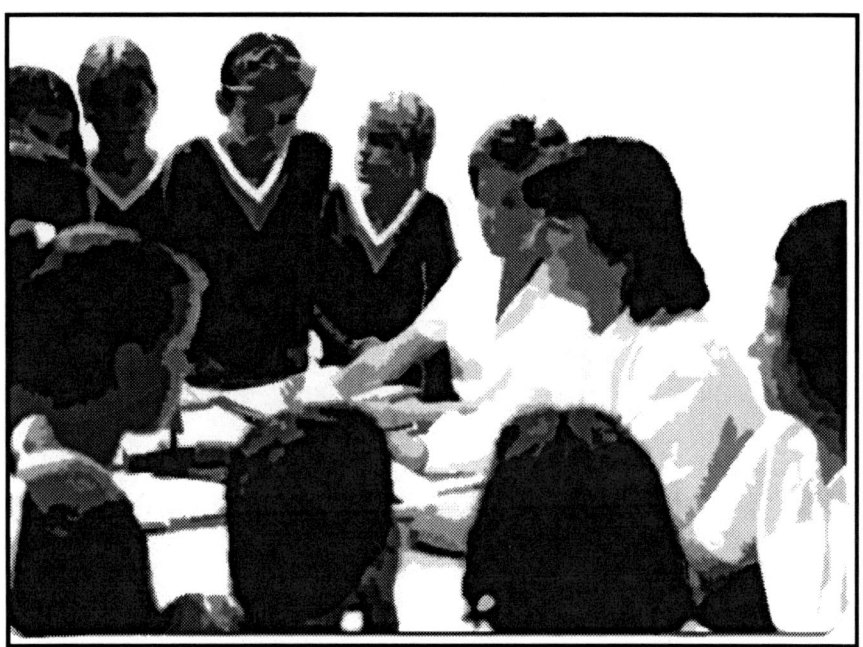

Competition

On the following pages are a few articles with information that may be helpful to you, especially if you are a first time competitor. In addition, the following pages have forms that allow you to track your scores at each meet (and other members of your competition rotation if you choose).

On the page opposite the score sheet, you can track the award(s) you earned on each event and record your feelings about each meet.

The bottom of the awards page is blank so you can draw, doodle, or paste stickers, pictures, or keepsakes from each competition.

Preparing for Competition: Eliminating Worry

Without a plan of action, you may find yourself worrying about minor details that can easily be taken care of before a competition.

Worrying, which is different from legitimate fear, is the inability to make a decision regarding a specific situation. Making a conscious choice for any situation will relax your mind and allow you to concentrate on what is important – the successful performance of your gymnastics routines.

Following are solutions to situations that may cause worry, which many a gymnast may face prior to a competition.

1. Travel and timing: Since you probably don't drive yet, your parents will need directions to the meet. Ask your coach for a map or written directions as well as open warm up times well in advance of the meet. Give the information to your parents – don't leave it in the bottom of your backpack or gym bag.

2. Preparation: The night before the meet, put everything you need in your gym bag. Ask your coach to review a list of necessities.

3. Waking up: You know your body and how long it takes you to "get it all together" in the morning. Wake up in plenty of time to be alert and focused for the competition. Get plenty of sleep the night before.

4. Nutrition: Eat early enough that your food is digested. Check with your coach and doctor for any special nutritional needs. If the competition is long, and hunger pangs develop, fruits, juices, and crackers are quickly assimilated by the body.

5. Warming up: Make sure you know your settings for uneven bars, vaulting, and beam. Stay focused and take advantage of your warm-up turns, since there may be several other gymnasts waiting in line. If you miss a skill, don't jump off and pout. Quickly remount and finish your turn. Remember, warm-ups don't necessarily predict what will happen in the meet, so don't get "psyched out" beforehand. If you spend most of your warm-up watching others perform, that means you aren't thinking about your own routines. Forget about everyone else.

6. Competition: Follow the rules of the competition and stay with your rotation. Avoid looking or talking to your parents or other spectators. Concentrate on your coach's instructions. Keep all of your competition gear safely inside your gym bag throughout the meet, unless you are currently using it.

7. Judges: Before and after each routine you are required to present yourself to the judges by saluting. When doing so, look the head judge directly in the eyes with a calm, confident expression. Regardless of what happens during the routine, never show your displeasure to the judges (or the audience) afterward. Even if you missed one of your skills, the judges may not have noticed if you covered well, but they will notice a bad attitude.

8. Scores: Remember, a score is not a judgment of you as an individual. It is an evaluation of a single gymnastics performance. Once you have completed a routine, leave it behind and concentrate on the next event.

9. Falls: If you should fall or have a major break in a routine, take the time to mentally prepare for the rest of the exercise. Check to see if you injured yourself. Chalk up again, if necessary. Once you are mentally composed, continue your routine as though you never had the break. It may be better to take a few extra moments to focus, regardless of a minor deduction. Consult with your coach.

10. Enjoy the moment. Above and beyond all the considerations listed above, learn how to enjoy yourself at meets. Lessons are learned in both success and failure. Remember the formula "Event + Response = Outcome." It's easy to enjoy the outcome when successful; the mark of a champion is learning to enjoy the process regardless of the outcome. Have fun at your next competition.

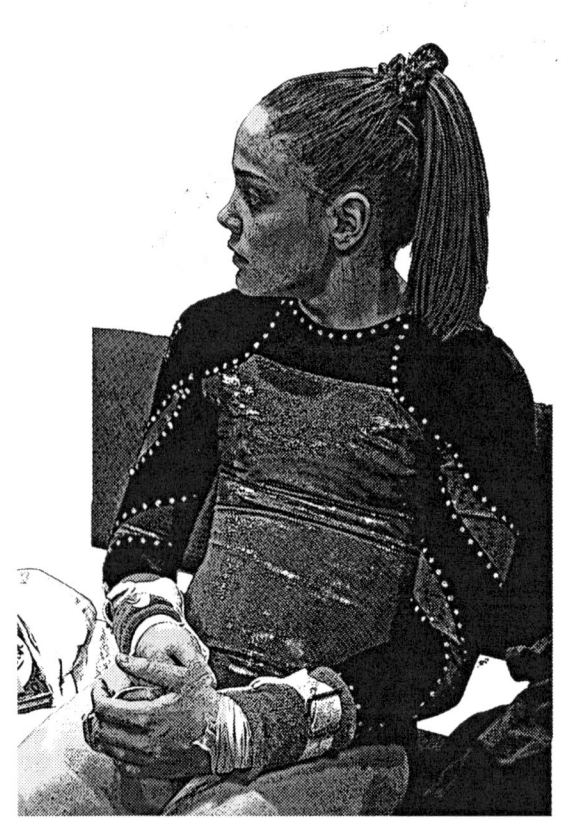

Gym bag necessities

At the end of your last practice before leaving for a competition, make sure the following items are in your gym bag:

- ☐ Uneven bar grips
    - o wrist wraps / gymnastics tape / pre-wrap
    - o hand lotion
    - o nail clippers
    - o alcohol wipes / soap / antibacterial spray
    - o Band-Aids.
- ☐ A copy of Compulsory / Optional Floor music on CD.
- ☐ Warm-up leotard (for hot climates / excess sweating).
- ☐ Team competition leotard.
- ☐ Team warm-up suit.
- ☐ Hair care
    - o Brush / Hair spray / Scrunchies
- ☐ Make-up, and personal hygiene items.
- ☐ Any vital medical braces, wrist supports, or bandages.
- ☐ Medical Release Form
    - o Necessary medicines
    - o Emergency phone numbers.
- ☐ Cell phone (turned off during meet!) or calling card.
- ☐ Money for meals on the road.
- ☐ Gymnastics Journal!
- ☐ Hand towel (especially when its hot).
- ☐ Water in unbreakable container (mostly necessary during hot/humid weather)
- ☐ Jump rope or Thera-band (to facilitate stretching exercises, cardiovascular work, and warm up drills).

Additional:

- ☐ Pen, leisure reading book, cards, Ipod/MP3, or video game (w/headphones).
- ☐ Fruit slices, juice, or crackers to snack on when the meet runs long (with coach's permission).

Meet etiquette for gymnasts

The following guidelines will help to make your competition fun as well as a rewarding experience.

- ❖ Be friendly and use sportsmanlike like conduct at all times.

Everybody has a unique way of experiencing gymnastics competition. Some people look for the fun in the experience; others are simply hoping to cope with their fears, while others are focused to the point of excluding everything else around them – including you!

This may at times make it seem difficult to be friendly with some gymnasts at a meet. Just remember, each gymnast is doing the best she is capable of at that moment.

When the opportunity presents itself, introduce yourself to the other gymnasts and coaches in your competitive rotation. Most of the time, you will have the chance to develop some new relationships, however, when another gymnast is being given directions by her coach or preparing to compete you must allow her time to concentrate without distraction.

- ❖ Stay focused on the competition. Talking with parents, relatives, or friends is inappropriate during the meet.

Even with the best of intentions, relatives and friends may give advice that conflicts with what your coach says. What will you do when you receive advice from Mom that differs from what Dad told you, and then the coach says something different? The answer is you will become more nervous and uptight because you do not know where to place your focus. During workouts and competition, you must listen only to your coach.

❖ Before leaving the competition floor, always inform your coach.

Always let your coach know when you are going to leave the competition floor. You don't want to miss your warm-up time or be missing when it is your turn to compete because you could get scratched from the meet.

In addition, never leave the competition facility or go to the parking lot without specific permission from your coach. You should always be accompanied by another team member or coach when leaving the competition floor. Also, let the coach know when you are leaving with your parents to go home so he/she knows everyone is safe.

❖ There is absolutely no reason for you to be on any piece of gymnastics equipment unless you are warming up or currently competing.

If you are staying to watch another teammate compete, or you have arrived early for warm ups, stay seated in the bleachers. Do not wander out onto the competition floor.

- Competing gymnasts must stay in their rotation group sitting quietly until the last competitor has finished.

- Gym bags, warm up suits, grips, and any other items you brought should be placed inside your gym bag and kept near you or under your chair.

- Warm ups or competition leotards should be worn when accepting awards - NO street clothes!

The meet is not complete until **ALL** the awards have been handed out. The other gymnasts have waited patiently to receive their awards and have applauded your efforts. You owe them the same consideration.

Safety at Competitions

Open warm-ups, timed-warm-ups, and even when you are on-deck to compete can present a few challenges to your personal safety at a gymnastics competition.

At a competition, everyone is focused on their own needs and tuning everything else out. In such a state of concentration, other gymnasts may walk right into your path as you prepare to tumble, or are running for a vault, or may even brush near a beam or walk under the bars! Obviously, this can cause distractions, potential falls or collisions – so keep your eyes and ears open to what is happening around you.

- In warm-ups, wait until your coach signals you the equipment is properly set before starting your routine.

- Keep an eye on people milling around the Vault runway. You may need to call out in a loud voice, **"VAULT!"** so they take notice and move away.

- On floor, make eye contact and be sure the other gymnasts understand you are next to tumble. Similar to Vault, call out **"TUMBLE!"** to get everyone's attention and let them know you want to perform a tumbling pass.

- On Bars and Beam your coach may keep meet helpers, like timers and set-up people out of the way, but gymnasts from other teams may still crowd you in their effort to make sure they get their fair share of warm-up time. Politely ask anyone encroaching on your workout space to move back.

Coaches have professional numbers, are safety certified, and most likely have the experience of attending several competitions, unlike volunteers who help to run the meet and may be on the floor with you. These helpers / volunteers may have little or no experience of the competitive situation so don't be surprised to find them standing in a dismount area, the middle of the vault runway, or struggling mightily at the judges table to get the stopwatch to work correctly. As with gymnasts, politely ask the to move from the workout area, however, leave them the dignity to figure out the stopwatch on their own.

Critical Attention Time

The most critical time to pay attention and watch for potential collisions is during a rotation from one event to another during warm-up (and possibly competition).

Some gymnasts are trying to take one last turn while other gymnasts are rushing to their next event to be first in line to take a turn. Coaches, gymnasts, and meet helpers may take shortcuts across workout areas assuming everybody is on the move. When traffic is in this condition, it may be best to move on to your next warm-up event.

"On Deck" Safety

"On Deck" means you are the next gymnast to compete at that event. Many gymnasts like to kick up to a handstand, do a bridge or back walkover to stretch their shoulders and back; some even do back handsprings and other skills off to the side of the equipment.

While this may be a "normal" occurrence at a meet, it may not be the safest thing to do on a hardwood or concrete floor. It may be better to warm-up dynamic skills in a properly matted area. Have one of your teammates standing by to direct traffic around you to prevent unexpected collisions. Remember, everyone is focused on her own routines and warm-up needs and may in fact be completely unaware of what you are doing until the moment of impact.

The Warm-Up Gym

Many gymnastics meets are expanding into mega-Invitational's with hundreds, if not thousands of competitors. In some instances, a gym separate from the competitive arena is set up for basic warm-up.

Unless a qualified gymnastics coach properly supervises you, it may not be a good idea to do anything other than basic stretches. Smaller gyms may have only one coach who may also need to be out on the competition floor. In those cases, you may want to ask your coach if another qualified coach will take the responsibility and supervise you during the open warm-up time.

Sometimes gymnasts and coaches forget that open warm-up is for stretching, not for doing routines or last-minute training of gymnastics skills. Using the excuse that other gymnasts are doing skills does not make it right for you to do it. If other gymnasts were licking the bottoms of their shoes, would you do that too? Probably not, so stay safe and use the warm-up gym for warming up only.

Sometimes spectators, especially younger brothers and sisters of competitors sneak away from mom and dad and find the warm-up gym, which is for them a wonderful playground, and give in to their natural urge to have fun. You may need to shoo them off the equipment for your safety and theirs.

For more information…

Overall, the quality of gymnastics competitions with USAG Sanctioning, Meet Director Certification, quality judging, and loads of information available through "Rules & Policies" among other publications available from USA Gymnastics[3] make competing in the sport of gymnastics a safe and enjoyable experience. Best of luck in your next competition.

---

[3] **www.usa-gymnastics.org**

Win, Lose, or Wipeout

It is important to remember that a score for any routine is an evaluation of one single performance in your career as a gymnast.

It is not a label you must live up to *(i.e. winning the all around this time means you must win it every time),* or hang around your neck for the rest of your life *(a 95th place ribbon for falling off the beam 20 times).*

Each meet teaches you more about your abilities as a gymnast, competitor, and human being, and provides the necessary ingredients for success at higher levels of competition.

Regardless of the outcome of a routine or overall competition, crying or feeling sorry for yourself is not an appropriate response to this situation or to most learning situations in the gym or normal life; neither is bragging about winning or pulling a superior attitude.

Learn to win generously, lose graciously, and always focus on developing your character. Hardly anybody will remember who won what within the next month, but they will remember how you treated them.

Treat others like the champion you are.

If you can't say anything nice to yourself…

Thought is the ancestor to every action you take. It doesn't matter whether you are peeling an orange or doing a double back somersault on floor. Your mind will work to achieve your currently dominant thought regardless of what it is; so think only about what you want.

Examples of self-talk:

"I'm a great dancer."

"I can't even boil water. I'm a terrible cook."

"I have a great bar routine."

"I always fall off once during my beam routine."

Whatever direction you give your mind; it will achieve. What you need to understand is the mind does not distinguish between negative and positive statements. It thinks in pictures. So, if your Mom says "Don't slam the car door!" All your mind sees is a picture of a car door slamming – and you slam the car door, even if you didn't mean to do it.

The basics of self-talk are:

1. Always state mentally and verbally what you want (to have, do, or be).

2. Adopt the posture and physicality of a person who is confident in achieving her goals.

3. Do your best on each attempt at your goals. Use the experience gained from each attempt to continually learn

and adapt your skills. (Note: If you achieve every goal on the first attempt, your goals are too easy. The fun in life comes from overcoming mistakes and learning from past failures.)

4. Change negatively oriented statements as soon as they occur. This will take continuous practice. We are all proficient in thinking of anything and everything that can go wrong. Be kind to yourself. You have had more than a few years of practicing negative self-talk. It will take at least a "few days" to substitute the old habit with the practice of goal/need/desire -oriented self-talk.

You don't always get what you want on each attempt, but in the long run, you usually get what you expect. Expect the best.

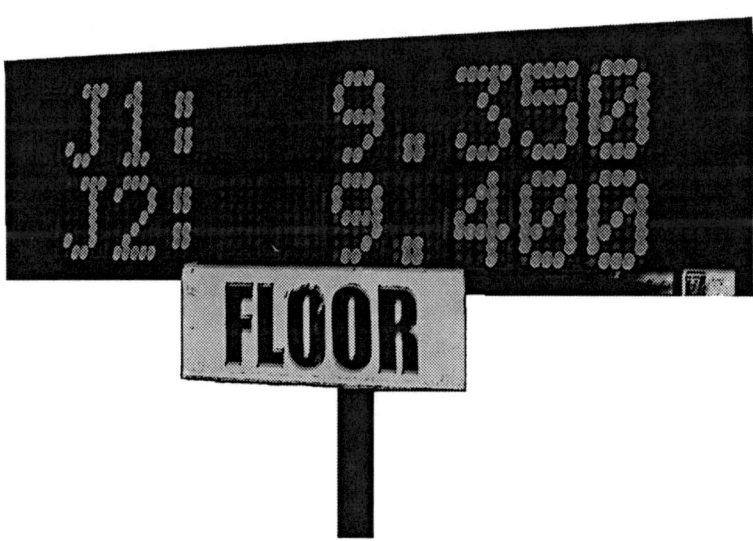

Meet Name: _____

Date: _____ **Time:** _____

City & State: _____

Name	Vault	Pl	Bars	Pl	Beam	Pl	Floor	Pl	AA	Pl

Meet Review

On **VAULT** I took _____ place.

On **BARS** I took _____ place.

On **BEAM** I took _____ place.

On **FLOOR** I took _____ place.

In the **ALL AROUND** I took _____ place.

The thing I would most like to improve or am proudest of on

VAULT is:_____.

BARS is:_____.

BEAM is:_____.

FLOOR is:_____.

The **BEST** thing about this meet is_____

_____

_____.

Pictures – Notes – Stickers:

Meet Name: _____

Date: _____ **Time:** _____

City & State: _____

Name	Vault	Pl	Bars	Pl	Beam	Pl	Floor	Pl	AA	Pl

Meet Review

On **VAULT** I took _____ place.

On **BARS** I took _____ place.

On **BEAM** I took _____ place.

On **FLOOR** I took_____ place.

In the **ALL AROUND** I took_____ place.

The thing I would most like to improve or am proudest of on

VAULT is:_____.

BARS is:_____.

BEAM is:_____.

FLOOR is:_____.

The **BEST** thing about this meet is_____

_____

_____.

Pictures – Notes – Stickers:

Meet Name:
Date: _____ Time: _____
City & State: _____

Name	Vault	Pl	Bars	Pl	Beam	Pl	Floor	Pl	AA	Pl

Meet Review

On **VAULT** I took _____ place.

On **BARS** I took _____ place.

On **BEAM** I took _____ place.

On **FLOOR** I took_____ place.

In the **ALL AROUND** I took_____ place.

The thing I would most like to improve or am proudest of on

VAULT is:_____.

BARS is:_____.

BEAM is:_____.

FLOOR is:_____.

The **BEST** thing about this meet is_____

_____

_____.

Pictures – Notes – Stickers:

Meet Name: _____

Date: _____ **Time:** _____

City & State: _____

Name	Vault	Pl	Bars	Pl	Beam	Pl	Floor	Pl	AA	Pl

Meet Review

On **VAULT** I took _____ place.

On **BARS** I took _____ place.

On **BEAM** I took _____ place.

On **FLOOR** I took_____ place.

In the **ALL AROUND** I took_____ place.

The thing I would most like to improve or am proudest of on

VAULT is:_____.

BARS is:_____.

BEAM is:_____.

FLOOR is:_____.

The **BEST** thing about this meet is_____

_____

_____.

Pictures – Notes – Stickers:

Meet Name: _____

Date: _____ **Time:** _____

City & State: _____

Name	Vault	Pl	Bars	Pl	Beam	Pl	Floor	Pl	AA	Pl

Meet Review

On **VAULT** I took _____ place.

On **BARS** I took _____ place.

On **BEAM** I took _____ place.

On **FLOOR** I took_____ place.

In the **ALL AROUND** I took_____ place.

The thing I would most like to improve or am proudest of on

VAULT is:_____.

BARS is:_____.

BEAM is:_____.

FLOOR is:_____.

The **BEST** thing about this meet is_____

_____

_____.

Pictures – Notes – Stickers:

Meet Name: _____

Date: _____ **Time:** _____

City & State: _____

Name	Vault	Pl	Bars	Pl	Beam	Pl	Floor	Pl	AA	Pl

Meet Review

On **VAULT** I took _____ place.

On **BARS** I took _____ place.

On **BEAM** I took _____ place.

On **FLOOR** I took _____ place.

In the **ALL AROUND** I took _____ place.

The thing I would most like to improve or am proudest of on

VAULT is:_____.

BARS is:_____.

BEAM is:_____.

FLOOR is:_____.

The **BEST** thing about this meet is_____

_____

_____.

Pictures – Notes – Stickers:

Meet Name:
Date: _____ Time: _____
City & State: _____

Name	Vault	Pl	Bars	Pl	Beam	Pl	Floor	Pl	AA	Pl

Meet Review

On **VAULT** I took _____ place.

On **BARS** I took _____ place.

On **BEAM** I took _____ place.

On **FLOOR** I took_____ place.

In the **ALL AROUND** I took_____ place.

The thing I would most like to improve or am proudest of on

VAULT is:_____.

BARS is:_____.

BEAM is:_____.

FLOOR is:_____.

The **BEST** thing about this meet is_____

_____

_____.

Pictures – Notes – Stickers:

Meet Name:
Date: _____ Time: _____
City & State: _____

Name	Vault	Pl	Bars	Pl	Beam	Pl	Floor	Pl	AA	Pl

Meet Review

On **VAULT** I took _____ place.

On **BARS** I took _____ place.

On **BEAM** I took _____ place.

On **FLOOR** I took_____ place.

In the **ALL AROUND** I took_____ place.

The thing I would most like to improve or am proudest of on

VAULT is:_____.

BARS is:_____.

BEAM is:_____.

FLOOR is:_____.

The **BEST** thing about this meet is_____

_____

_____.

Pictures – Notes – Stickers:

Meet Name: _____

Date: _____ **Time:** _____

City & State: _____

Name	Vault	Pl	Bars	Pl	Beam	Pl	Floor	Pl	AA	Pl

Meet Review

On **VAULT** I took _____ place.

On **BARS** I took _____ place.

On **BEAM** I took _____ place.

On **FLOOR** I took_____ place.

In the **ALL AROUND** I took_____ place.

The thing I would most like to improve or am proudest of on

VAULT is:_____.

BARS is:_____.

BEAM is:_____.

FLOOR is:_____.

The **BEST** thing about this meet is_____

_____

_____.

Pictures – Notes – Stickers:

Meet Name: _____

Date: _____ **Time:** _____

City & State: _____

Name	Vault	Pl	Bars	Pl	Beam	Pl	Floor	Pl	AA	Pl

Meet Review

On **VAULT** I took _____ place.

On **BARS** I took _____ place.

On **BEAM** I took _____ place.

On **FLOOR** I took _____ place.

In the **ALL AROUND** I took _____ place.

The thing I would most like to improve or am proudest of on

VAULT is:_____.

BARS is:_____.

BEAM is:_____.

FLOOR is:_____.

The **BEST** thing about this meet is_____

_____

_____.

Pictures – Notes – Stickers:

Meet Name: _____

Date: _____ **Time:** _____

City & State: _____

Name	Vault	Pl	Bars	Pl	Beam	Pl	Floor	Pl	AA	Pl

Meet Review

On **VAULT** I took _____ place.

On **BARS** I took _____ place.

On **BEAM** I took _____ place.

On **FLOOR** I took _____ place.

In the **ALL AROUND** I took _____ place.

The thing I would most like to improve or am proudest of on

VAULT is:_____.

BARS is:_____.

BEAM is:_____.

FLOOR is:_____.

The **BEST** thing about this meet is_____

_____

_____.

Pictures – Notes – Stickers:

Meet Name: _____

Date: _____ **Time:** _____

City & State: _____

Name	Vault	Pl	Bars	Pl	Beam	Pl	Floor	Pl	AA	Pl

Meet Review

On **VAULT** I took _____ place.

On **BARS** I took _____ place.

On **BEAM** I took _____ place.

On **FLOOR** I took_____ place.

In the **ALL AROUND** I took_____ place.

The thing I would most like to improve or am proudest of on

VAULT is:_____.

BARS is:_____.

BEAM is:_____.

FLOOR is:_____.

The **BEST** thing about this meet is_____

_____

_____.

Pictures – Notes – Stickers:

A-maze-ing Goals

The maze below is like a metaphor for gymnastics. Very few people make it through the maze in one attempt. A path is blocked, you have to back track, you need to turn right instead of left, and there may be more than one route to your goal.

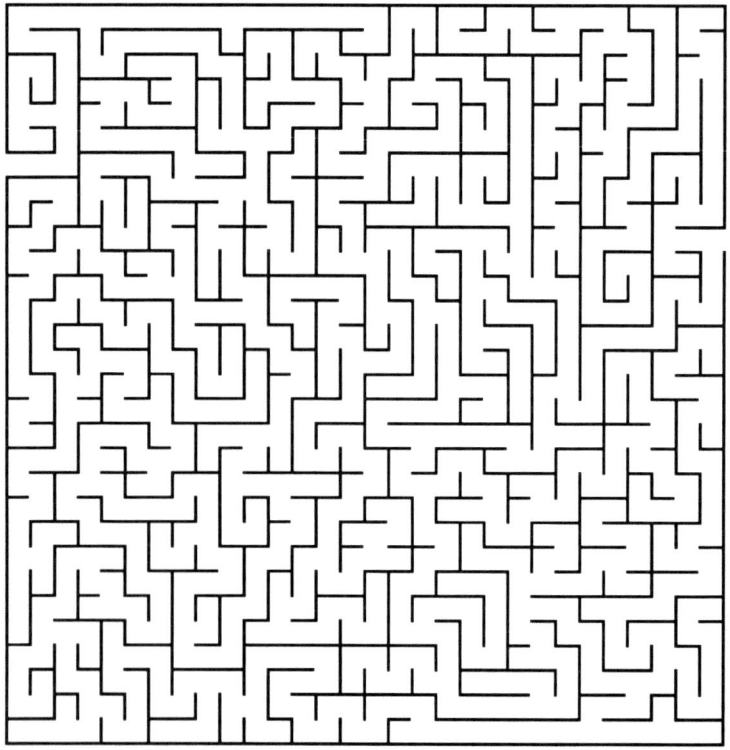

The same is true in workouts, competition, and life. If one path does not lead to your goal, there are still plenty of other paths.

Hint: Parents, teachers, and coaches have been through the maze many times and are here to help guide you. While the mazes they have walked to reach their goals may have been different, they are experienced travelers / goal-seekers who can make helpful suggestions to guide you to success.

Gymnastics Anagrams – unscramble the words.

Clue											
Am clean babe	b	a	l	a	n	c	e	b	e	a	m
Menace a blab											
Fixes core role											
A snub nerve											
All but a vet											
Unwary											
Drops in brag											
Neat Lamp											
Mint tags											
A red lot											
Ha! X block											
bolt stock ping											
In and slouching											
Search self or…											
Add shag run											

Word Search: Gymnasts (1)

```
S A N O S N H O J Y D N A R B Y L L U
L V I D A A S A R I V L E O T B G U M M
L R E R Q Z V I V P I N J U N D D N K I
I W S T C Y X I M O O T K S Y M B A C K
M P E V L K D B L S T L X Z I M U E E E
E A T N D A P H N I P A M L I W N R L I
B T R Y D R N H M E S I L C Z A N U I L
E U A N D Y O A X O Y A H I M G Q G B L
O B C M A J B U B H T E L O F J P N A E
H R E T Y G A R D O L V C E D A C U L N
P O E H U J N E U L G A A O I H I A E Z
P K T D Y F M R E C I I Y L J N H R M A
C A A X R R I D P D E M N M D D A O A M
K G L S Y S U F A X W K J S Z B P D P M
Q L A U C S B N Y C V X R J K U X O L G
X O V H S A V O N U H S U H S A N E L E
M X E E J I Z C A T H Y R I G B Y T P B
Z V R X E P N O T T E R U O L Y R A M W
A R A M A N C M E N N A I L U J D I X Y
E A H I B X L T I R G W M Z K V X C A A
```

BRANDY JOHNSON
CATHY RIGBY
DANIELA SILIVAS
ELENA SHUSHUNOVA
ELVIRA SAADI
JULIANNE MCNAMARA
KATHY JOHNSON
LUDMILLA TOURISCHEVA
MARIA FILATOVA
MARY LOU RETTON
MICHELLE DUSSERRE
NADIA COMANECI
NELLIE KIM
OLGA KORBUT
PAMELA BILECK
PHOEBE MILLS
SVETLANA BOGINSKAYA
TEODORA UNGUREANU
TRACEE TALAVERA
WENDY BRUCE

(Coloring Page[4])

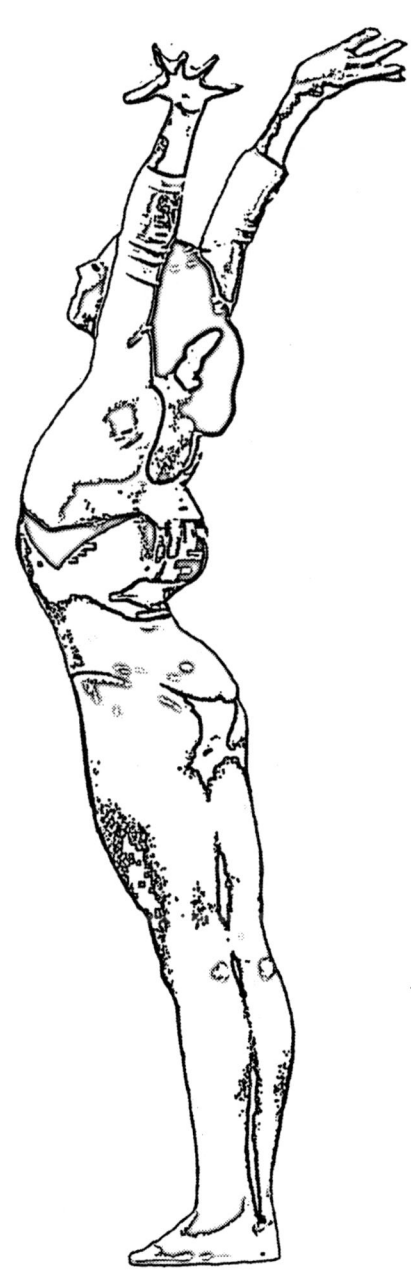

---
[4] **Warning: Use colored pencils only. Felt tip markers may bleed through to the other side of the page.**

Word Search: Fruits

```
G H S T R A W B E R R I E S J
K Y E P U O L A T N A C T Q D
T T I P L G N S N I S I A R H
J B R A B U L Z A Y U N N W C
I D R P L E M S S R A P A M A
C H E R R I E S F N J T R S E
O O B E S T Y E A N E T G F P
F N K R A S P B E R R I E S A
Y E C D P A O C M T F U M O P
O Y A Z R G T E G N A R O L A
D D L G R A L H V C B F P E Y
K E B A R O Z S T O C I R P A
O W P I N E A P P L E W L N H
A E N I R E G N A T Y I U P M
S E N U R P O G N A M K M J H
```

APPLE
APRICOTS
BANANA
BLACKBERRIES
CANTALOUPE
CHERRIES
DATES
FIGS
GRAPEFRUIT
GRAPES
HONEYDEW
KIWIFRUIT
MANGO
NECTARINE
ORANGE
PAPAYA
PEACH
PINEAPPLE
PLUMS
POMEGRANATE
PRUNES
RAISINS
RASPBERRIES
STRAWBERRIES
TANGERINE
WATERMELON

(Coloring Page[5])

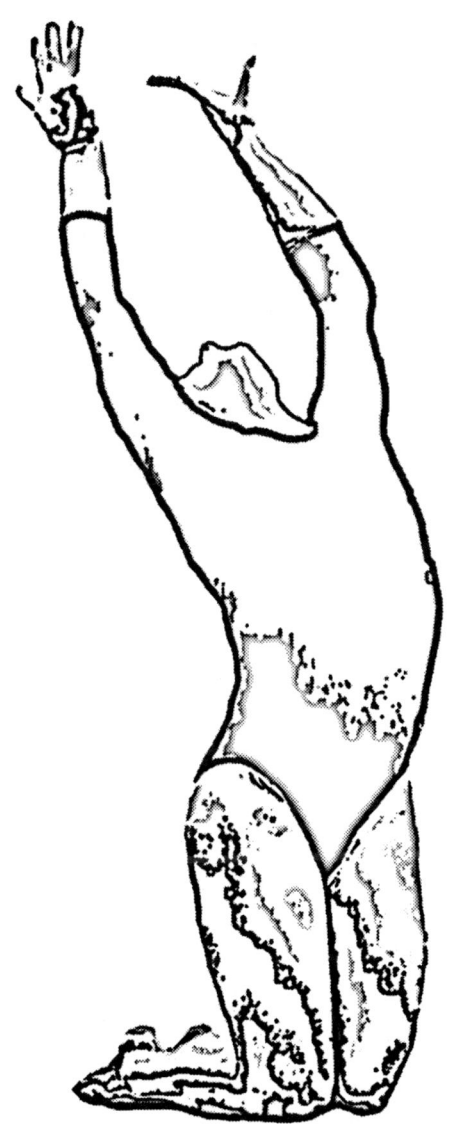

---
[5] Warning: Use colored pencils only. Felt tip markers may bleed through to the other side of the page.

Word Search: Gymnastics

```
Y O D L X Z R E H S A L F E R O C S H V
A R N Y B S I P G U N L E X L Z Y T A R
Y P U M R A W N E P O J N Y I X A H Y E
Y R O D A C L H J O I E M L N M W B G D
Z V R L E O T A R D T P V T L Q N D B Q
S R A B N E V E N U I T I E A P U N K B
X T L N Z E X B K C T M N D N J R G H S
P N L I C E Y D O Y E A D R D T Y I T L
D U A H R F A R R D P B Y A I M A I H K
C O A C H T D V W A M R E W N Q N X B A
F M I R E E N A O Q O H C A G G W C A Z
A S I A R E R U R T C B S H M I B D K V
E I U M J M T L A V E T G A A Q C X I I
K D C Q U S I T A V I Q T N T L N A O N
U M N P X V I T F C X B Y V I L K N Q R
F P Q O H O K A S K R S C U N R N B U I
F Z E E N Y Y B X H W Q T O A M P M O O
P N N F E T U L A S K R J C W M P S M X
S Y N O M E R E C F A D N T X C Z K W S
Z J O Y G T Z B X V S J X K P H T N S S
```

ALL AROUND
AWARD
BALANCE BEAM
CEREMONY
CHALK BOX
COACH
COMPETITION
DISMOUNT
EVENT
FLOOR EXERCISE
GYMNASTICS
HEAD JUDGE
LANDING MAT
LEOTARD
MARCH IN

MEET FEE
MOUNT
OLYMPIC ORDER
OPEN WARM UP
PANEL MAT
ROTATION
RUNWAY
SALUTE
SCORE FLASHER
SPRINGBOARD
STING MAT
TIMED WARM UP
UNEVEN BARS
VAULT TABLE

(Coloring Page[6])

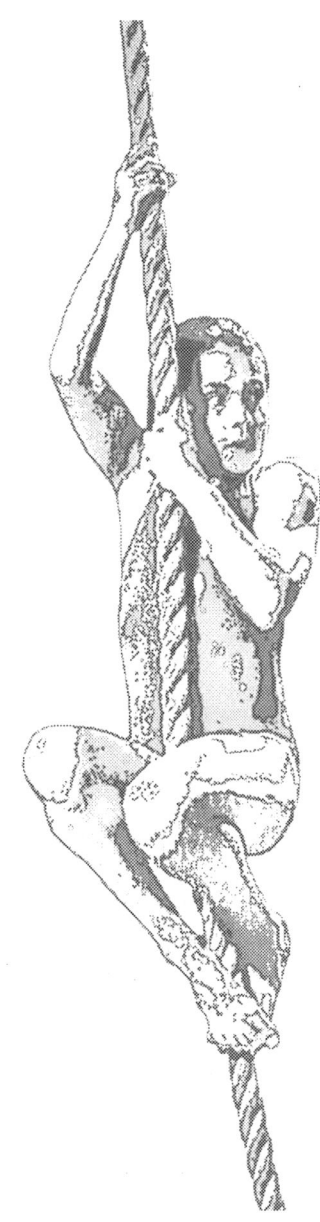

---
[6] **Warning: Use colored pencils only. Felt tip markers may bleed through to the other side of the page.**

Word Search: Vegetables

```
W V S N A E B C A R R O T S D
R Q Q U B G W M I S C P E A S
A S P A R A G U S D Z O N V S
D A E Z U B O S P R T D T S R
I U O T S B K H K A E R U Q E
S E K N S A R R M L F A R U B
H R L A E C A O I L H T N A M
E K E L L M T O C O X S I S U
S R T P S E N M C C W U P H C
N A T G P G J S L C O M S C U
O U U G R E W O L F I L U A C
I T C E O K P Z U C C H I N I
N N E F U E N D I V E H F I B
O N W U T C E L E R Y O S P I
S P C O S P I N S R A P G S K
```

ASPARAGUS
BEANS
BROCCOLI
BRUSSEL SPROUTS
CABBAGE
CARROTS
CAULIFLOWER
CELERY
COLLARDS
CUCUMBERS
DANDELION GREENS

EGGPLANT
ENDIVE
KALE
LETTUCE
MUSHROOMS
MUSTARD
OKRA
ONIONS
PARSNIPS
PEAS
PEPPERS

RADISHES
REDPEPPERS
SAUERKRAUT
SPINACH
SPROUTS
SQUASH
TOMATOES
TURNIPS
ZUCCHINI

(Coloring Page[7])

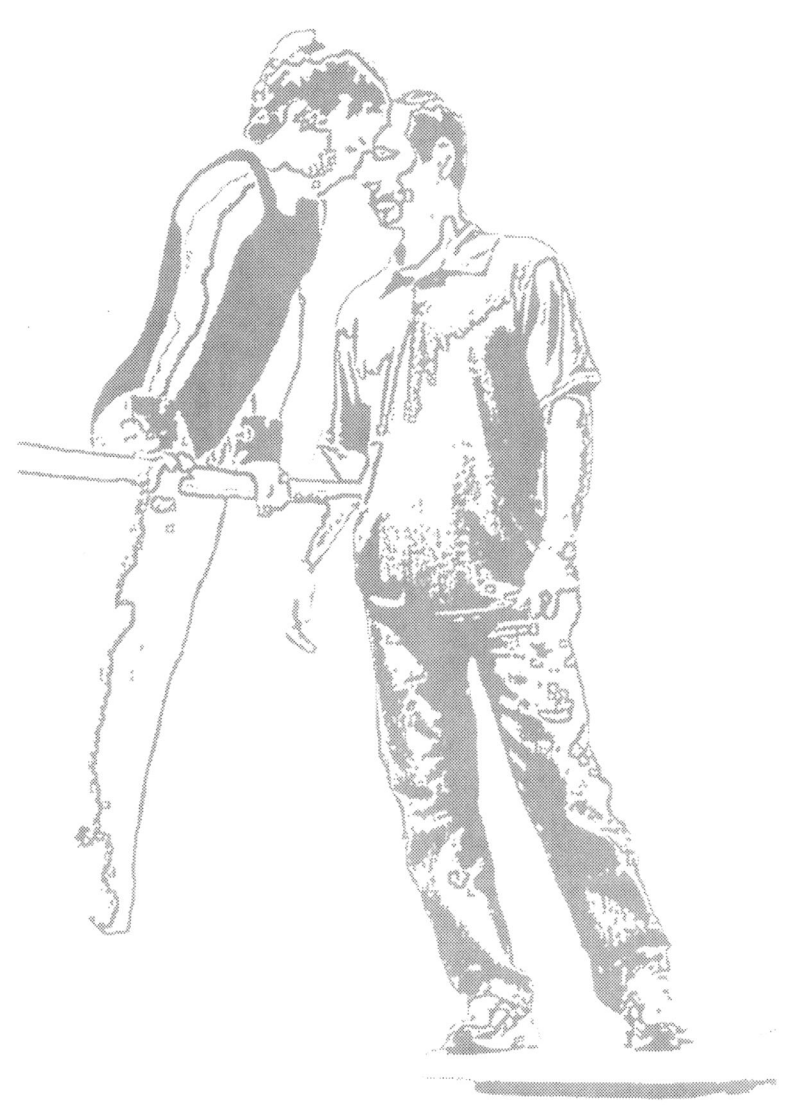

---

[7] **Warning: Use colored pencils only. Felt tip markers may bleed through to the other side of the page.**

Word Search: Gymnasts (2)

```
Z A K E L D V D K K D S I I S D I A P D
Q S R X M I A O Q H G H E R O C J N J D
S T E X O G L M Q V F B O M I C S I R G
S P L E H P E I C Y A J I V V I C K U M
G N L R O L J N A C C N O Q P A K R S O
L E I H D G R I D P I S B D R M T O T H
H D M K V J Y Q M Q O B Y L T S S H M I
K R N U Q G O U U L D D Y E I X T K U N
I O O B X S V E I X Q P K R W N E A M I
M B N D Y X D M A R A X R O I T P N V B
Z A N Z A A A O I T M E B R P W U A K H
M D A Y W I O C T C K N M M Q A K L X A
E N H E N R I E T T A Ó N O D I Y T G R
S A S I N U R A X D N H J K C L E E E D
K M V B Y S M N T H H C E O D V N V V W
A A I F O Y S U L O M I P F G B T S T A
L K H N C K Y E R H P M U H N I R E T J
R W L H N R B L G R P K V R W G U N I Z
T Q O E C O U R T N E Y M C C O O L W H
Z W P O P C J B W G J B B H N C C O A Z
```

AMANDA BORDEN
AMY CHOW
CARLY PATTERSON
COURTNEY KUPETS
COURTNEY MCCOOL
DOMINIQUE DAWES
DOMINIQUE MOCEANU
HENRIETTA ÓNODI
JAYCIE PHELPS
KERRI STRUG
KIM ZMESKAL
LAVINIA MILOSOVICI
LILIA PODKOPAYEVA
MOHINI BHARDWAJ
SHANNON MILLER
SVETLANA KHORKINA
TERIN HUMPHREY

(Design a leotard [8])

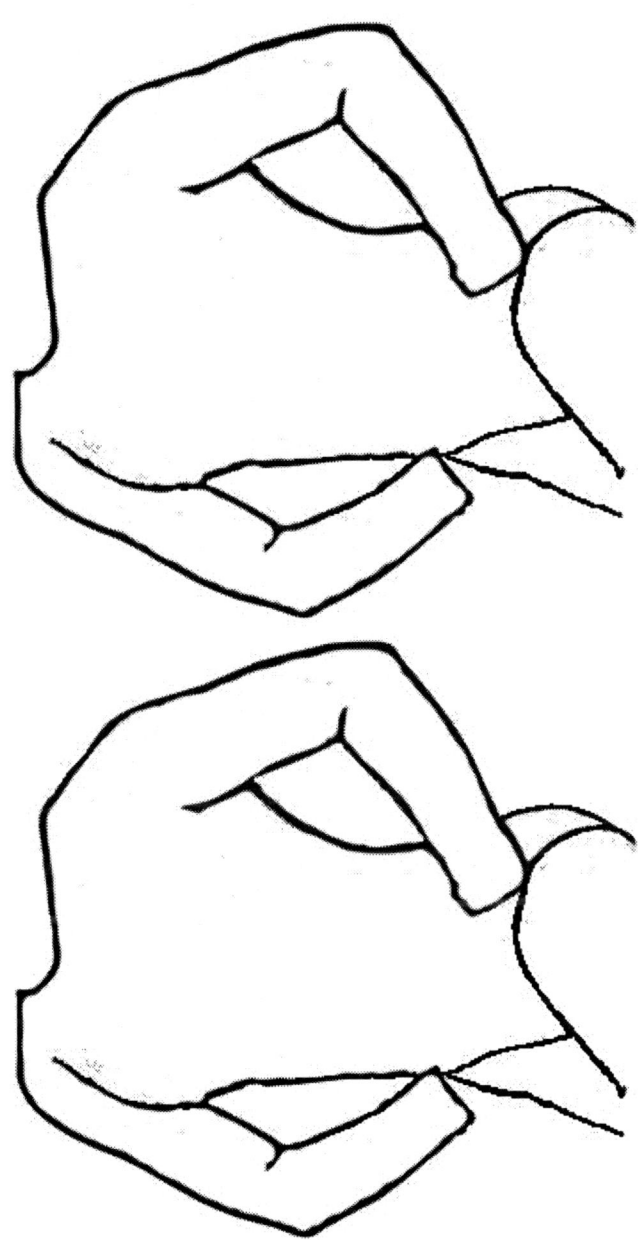

[8] Warning: Use colored pencils only. Felt tip markers may bleed through to the other side of the page.

Gymnastics Anagrams – unscramble the words.

Felt puff hit
Church is yarn
Tighter liar
Pride glows
Stigma by gem
Jaded huge
Outer brain
Blast impugns
Tame best hop
Notoriety soup
Up manpower!
Matured wimp
I'm not poetic
Foul on rioter
I am true bone

(Design a leotard [9])

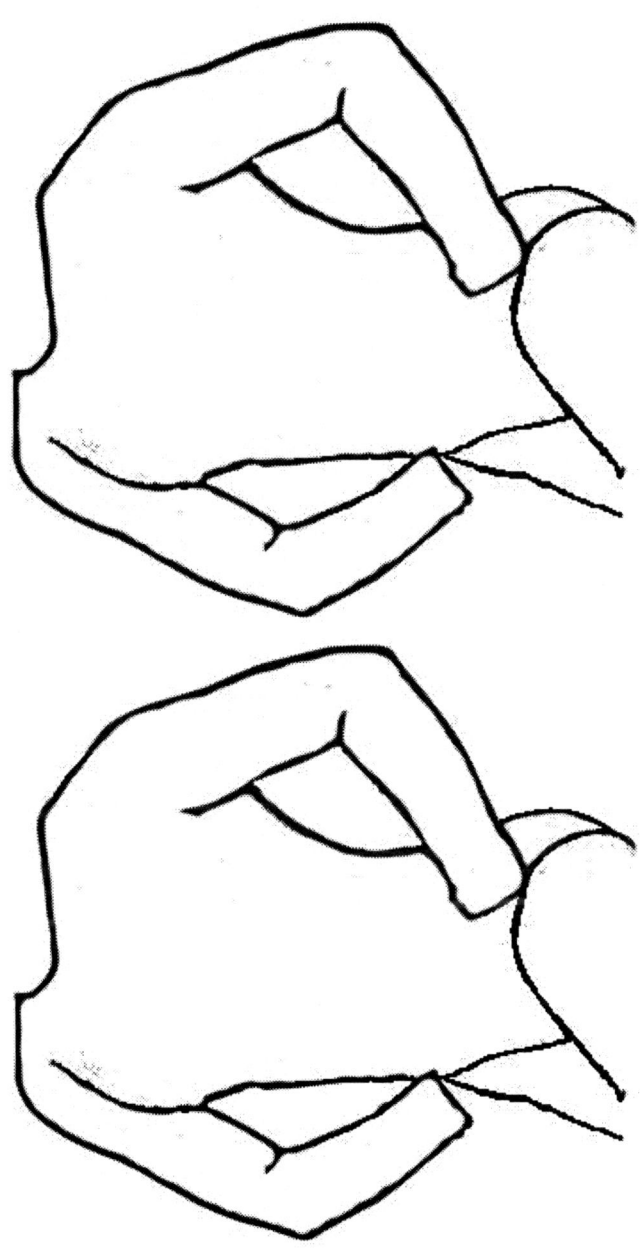

---
[9] **Warning: Use colored pencils only. Felt tip markers may bleed through to the other side of the page.**

Extended Tic-Tac-Toe

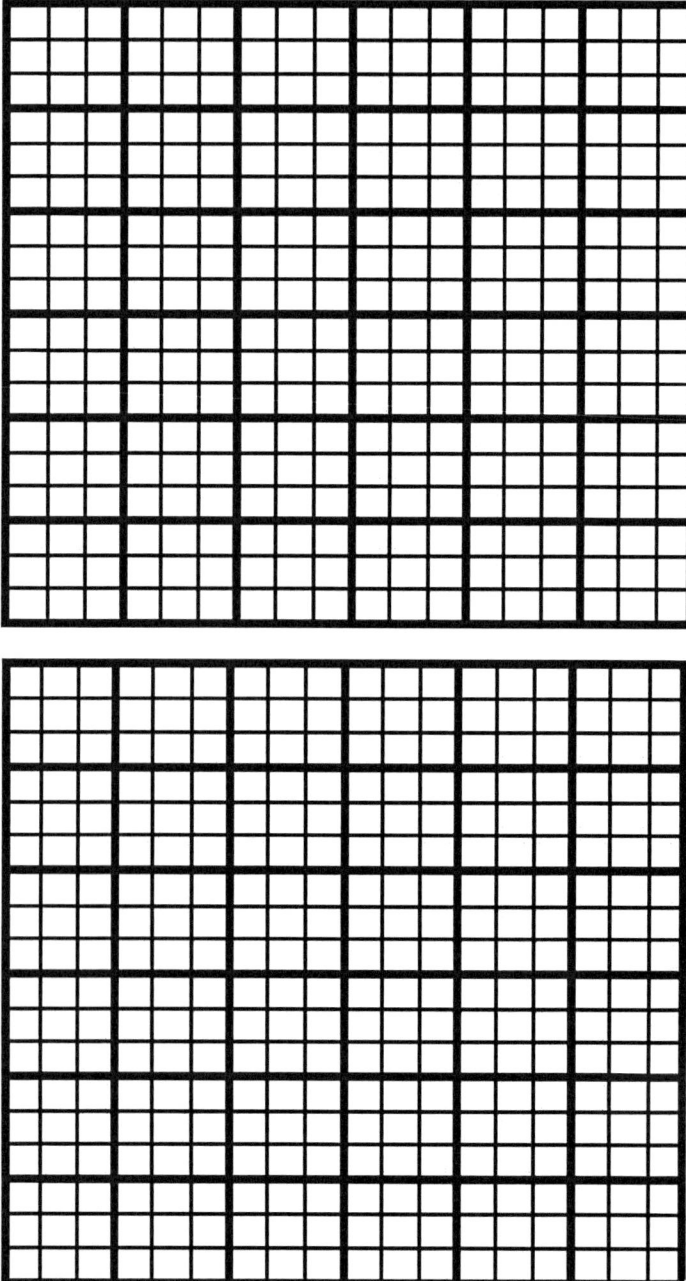

Each 3x3 grid is a single game of tic-tac-toe, however, you can extend the game giving points for each **X** or **O** that is connected in a straight or diagonal line through multiple grids.

Extended Tic-Tac-Toe

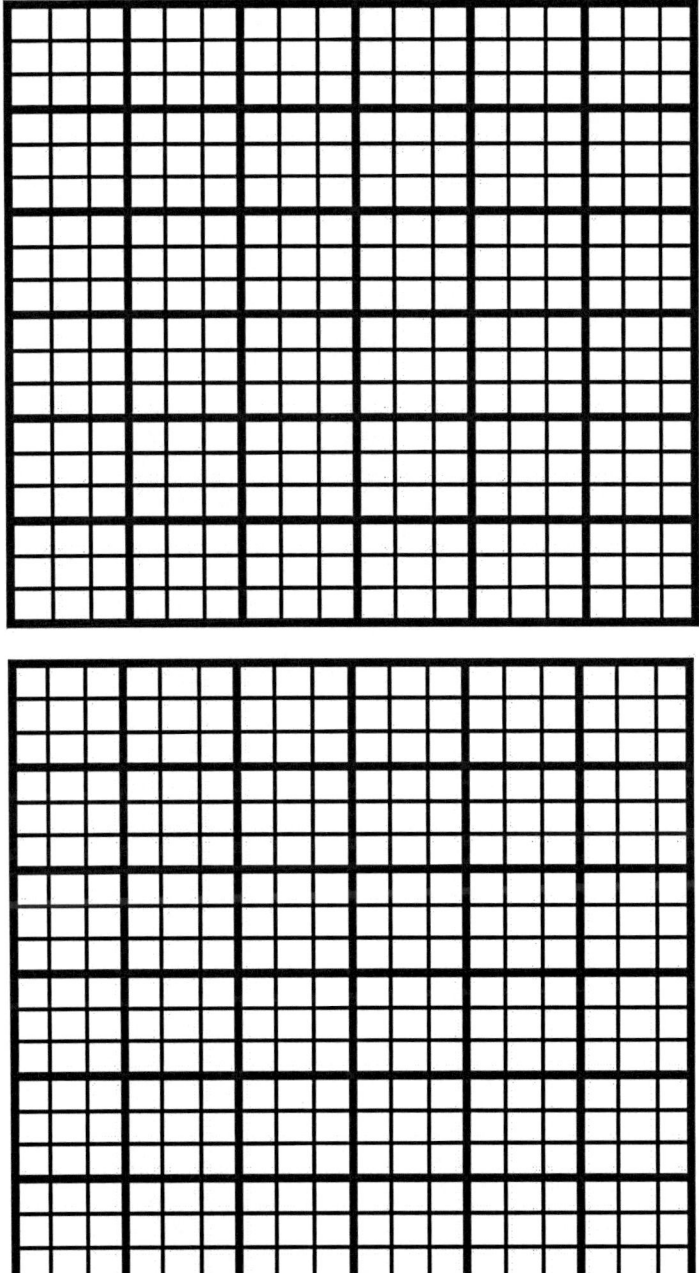

Autographs

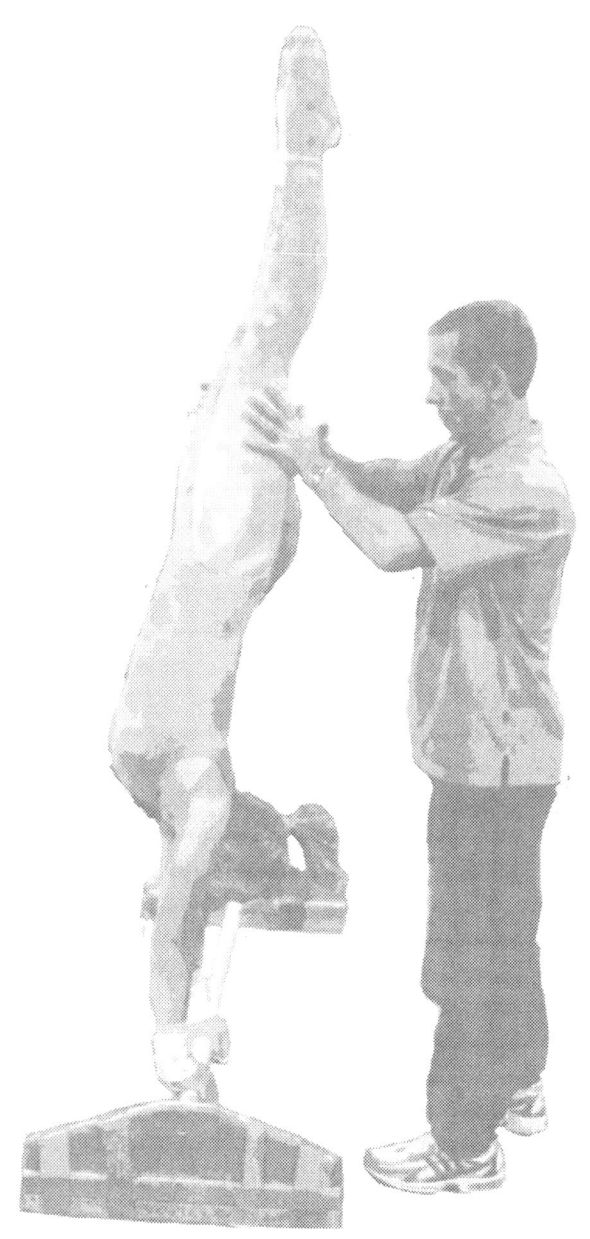

Autographs

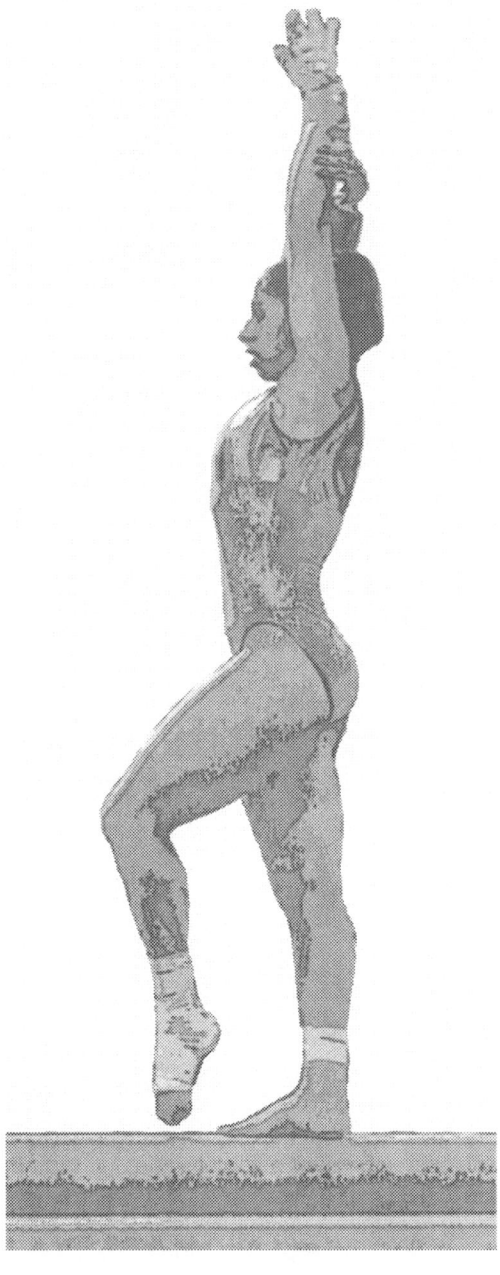

Vision Page [10]

---

[10] On these "Vision Pages", the idea is for you to paste pictures, drawings, icons, photographs – anything that represents your currently dominant goal(s). Look at, daydream, and visualize the goals represented here as often as possible, preferably using as many senses as possible (seeing, touching, hearing, smelling, tasting, and feeling emotionally) in dynamic or moving mental pictures.

Vision Page

Address / phone / email

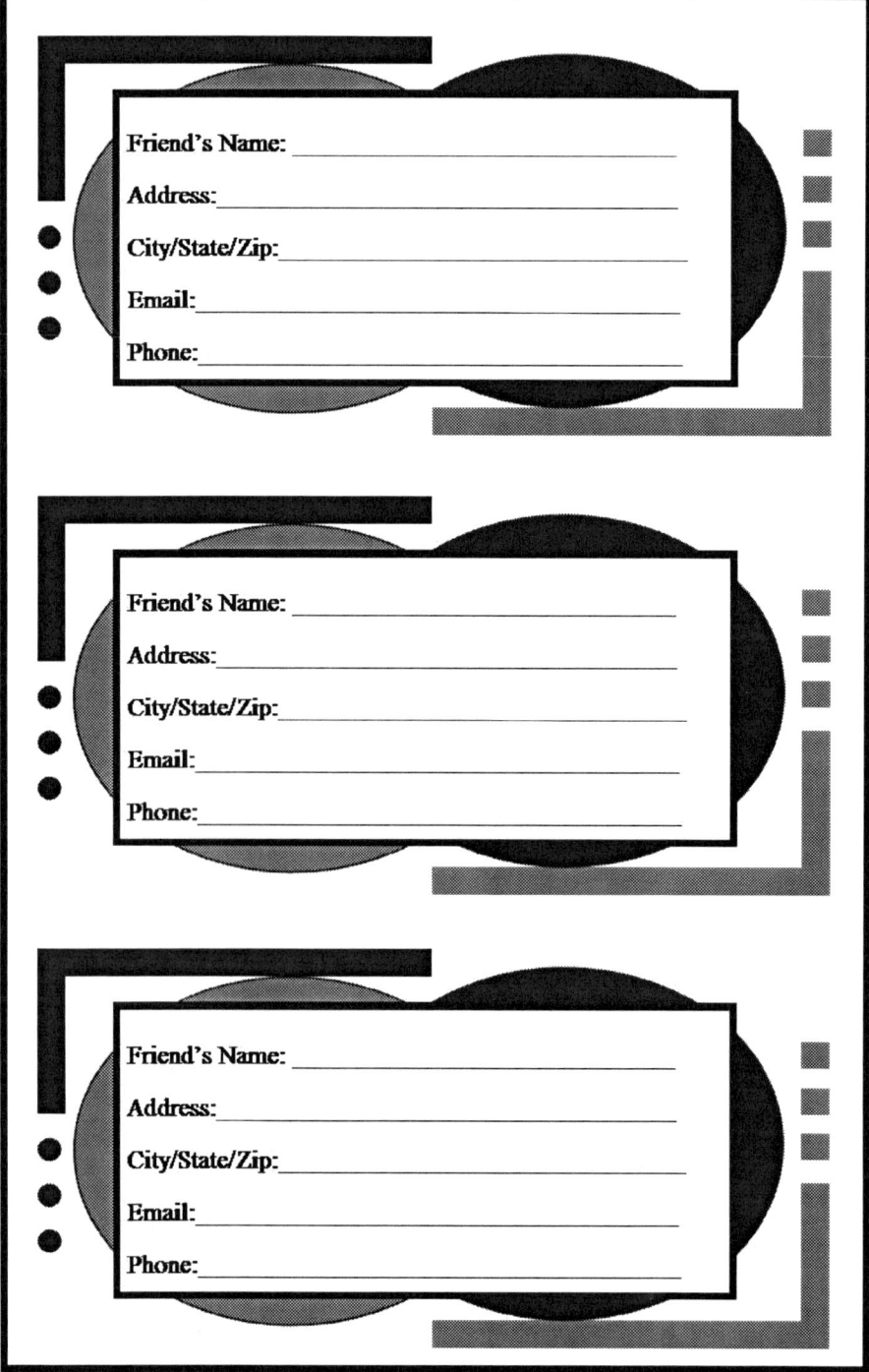

Friend's Name: _____
Address: _____
City/State/Zip: _____
Email: _____
Phone: _____

Friend's Name: _____
Address: _____
City/State/Zip: _____
Email: _____
Phone: _____

Friend's Name: _____
Address: _____
City/State/Zip: _____
Email: _____
Phone: _____

Address / phone / email

Friend's Name: _____
Address: _____
City/State/Zip: _____
Email: _____
Phone: _____

Friend's Name: _____
Address: _____
City/State/Zip: _____
Email: _____
Phone: _____

Friend's Name: _____
Address: _____
City/State/Zip: _____
Email: _____
Phone: _____

Address / phone / email

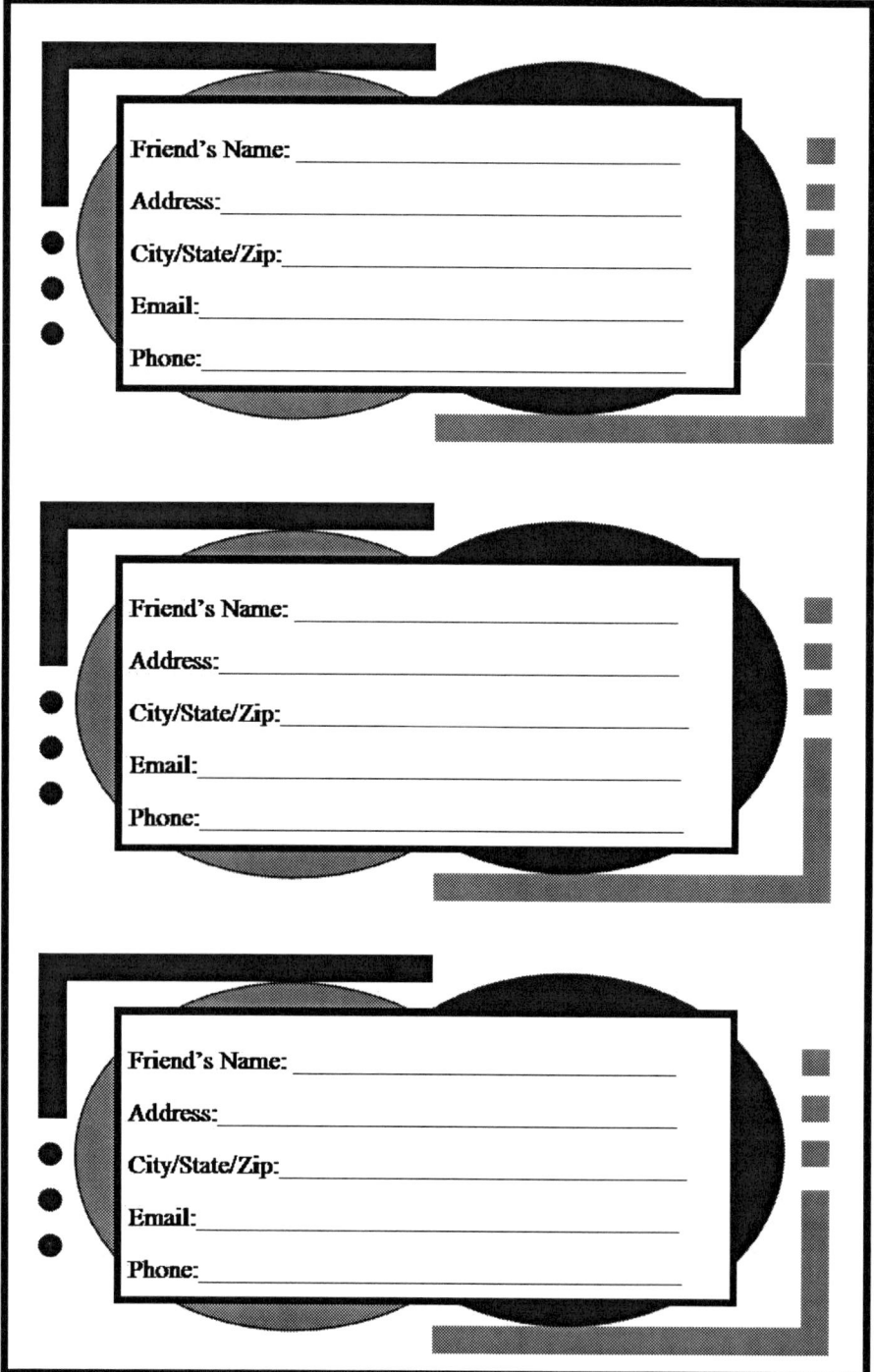

Friend's Name: _____
Address: _____
City/State/Zip: _____
Email: _____
Phone: _____

Friend's Name: _____
Address: _____
City/State/Zip: _____
Email: _____
Phone: _____

Friend's Name: _____
Address: _____
City/State/Zip: _____
Email: _____
Phone: _____

Make a Choice

Make a Choice;
reach a Decision;
take some Action;
with no chance of Revision.

In your effort to Create;
you may stumble over Fate;
patiently burn with the Need
to have, do, be, - Succeed!

Relieve the stress of Indecision
that takes a mental Toll;
stoke the flames of Desire
with a plan to reach your Goal.

The key to Success
is in personal Inquisition;
reinforced and Supported
by a strong mental Vision.

Coincidence and Synchronicity;
stem from the Law of Attraction.
A confident belief in your Choice
that delivers ultimate Satisfaction.

Make a Choice;
reach a Decision;
take some Action;
with no chance of Revision.
The Law of Attraction
rewards consistent Vision.

- Rik Feeney

Printed in the United States
77205LV00001B/1-60